Your Secret Chamber

Written and developed by Diana Anderson
Ketchum, Idaho
Copyright © 2012 Diana Anderson

Published by Words as My Wings, LLC
All Rights Reserved

ISBN-13: 978-0-9853307-0-5
ISBN-10: 0-9853307-0-8
First Addition Printed March 2012

Printed in the United States

Table of Contents

Five Weeks of Pleasure

WEEK #1

Introduction: Straight Talk on Sex

    How to take this course

    What this book is designed to do

    Who will be helped by this workbook?

Chapter 1: Benefits of Sex and Orgasm

    Where is your secret chamber?

    Twenty-four ways that sex provides better physical, emotional & mental health

Chapter 2: Hang-ups about Sex

    Overcoming fears, doubts and judgments about sex

Chapter 3: Let Your Man Love You.

How to break the walls down that keep love and intimacy away

WEEK #2

Chapter 4: Let Your Man See You

How to feel sexy when you're naked

What makes you feel sexy and sexually aroused?

Chapter 5: Learning to Blossom:

Becoming mentally and physically available

Trust, feeling desirable, feeling present with your partner, feeling cared for, and self-care

WEEK #3

Chapter 6: Being Present

Connecting with your partner

Communicating about pleasure

WEEK #4

Chapter 7: Arousal is the Key to Pleasure

There are many different ways to get aroused

Know your body and what brings you pleasure

Chapter 8: Let's Talk Orgasm

    How to achieving many types of orgasms.

WEEK #5

Chapter 9: Allowing the Deepest Penetration

    Once you trust your partner, surrender your body to him, open your heart,
your throat, your labia and vagina

Chapter 10: Don't Get Caught

    Avoiding STD's

Resources:

    Quick Reference page

    My seminars

    My website

    Other Amazon Books by this author:

- *Always in the Mood*
- *Deep Connection*

    Coming In February 2013:

- *Manifesting with Passion*

Drawing of Female Anatomy of Reproductive System

About the Author

Grab the whole The Venus Method Series:

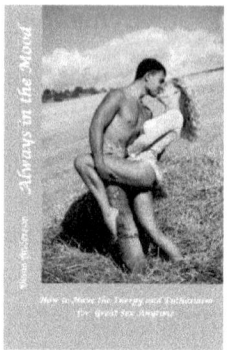

Always in the Mood; A powerful booklet about how to feel ready for your man when he desires you, and enjoy his approach, for great intimacy anytime.

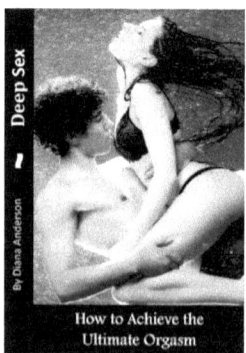

Deep Sex: How to Achieve your Ultimate Orgasm

All orgasms are not created equally. The art of the female climax, long shrouded in mystery and elusive for many women, is made accessible in this down-to-earth, illuminating text. Author and intimacy coach, Diana Anderson presents the essential ingredients and chemistry necessary to achieve advanced orgasmic experience and deep connection with your partner.

http://www.amazon.com/-/e/B00AQ5P61W

http:/www.amazon.com/-/e/B00AQ5P61W

Your Secret Chamber

How to take this course:

This course is designed to be more than a book. It is an instruction manual to guide you from a place of limitations in sexuality, and in life, to a place of limitless pleasure and infinite expression of the self.

First, follow the chapters in order. Each chapter builds on the other. It is also crucial to complete the sexercises in each chapter. Without practice, you won't get better. If you read this book from cover to cover, without practicing, nothing will change for you. Getting good takes practice.

Please get a journal to write about your experience with the sexercises and what you might do to improve next time, or print this book out and write on the workbook pages. It will seem very foreign at first to write about sexual experiences. You may be afraid that someone will find your journal. Part of opening up sexually is learning to talk about and write about sex without being ashamed. It is completely freeing. It takes the secrets and taboos out of sex and brings it into the natural light of organic, wholesome pleasure.

Your Secret Chamber

There is nothing to hide from yourself or your partner in regards to sexuality. You are born to have and enjoy sex. If you follow each chapter, this book will change how you perceive sex and how much you enjoy it.

What this course is designed to do for you.

The goals of this Sexercise book are:

1. To take you step by step to a cosmic, ecstatic level of orgasm
2. To make you crave more love making
3. To open you up to your full authentic, creative, feminine expression
4. To empower you to treasure and use the colossal energy that your orgasms produce
5. Improve your intimate relationship through better sex and bonding
6. Guide you to be more deeply penetrated by your lover so that he can access hidden levels you haven't found on your own and unlock the doors to your authentic inner-beauty and creativity.
7. Teach you how to allow the masculine energy to open you up
8. Help you reach the best orgasms of your life
9. Awaken energy in your body and allow that energy to move more freely

Questions and Answers

Your Secret Chamber

Who Benefits from the Course?

You may be asking yourself, will this course have any value to me? Below are questions you might ask before deciding if you want to use this workbook.

Before we begin here, let me mention that my first goal is to help you loosen up in regards to sex. In working towards that goal, I have made this book a bit risqué and littered with sex words to help you "get over it". If you want the best orgasms of your life, you have to let go and open up to the big, wide-world of sex. So, for your benefit, I'm holding nothing back.

1. **I have regular orgasms. They are usually pretty good. Why should I read a course on orgasms?**
   This workbook is about achieving better and better orgasms. The level that you can achieve is limitless, always able to be improved upon. This workbook consists of step by step exercises to improve your orgasms and take you to, or build you towards having the best orgasm possible.

Your Secret Chamber

Opening to more sexual pleasure opens you up to more authentic expression, as well as more vitality and improved health.

2. **I am unable to have orgasms. I don't even know if they are real. Can this workbook help me?**

There are many reasons why you may not be having orgasms. This manual can help:

a. If you don't understand the physical elements of your body and how to become aroused
b. If you are not in touch with the sensations of your body
c. If you don't know how to feel open and connected with your lover
d. If you are stuck in your head
e. If you are inexperienced

I will lead you step by step through all of the issues above.

However, if your difficultly with orgasm is a physical impairment, or from emotional trauma, such as unhealed sexual abuse, this book is not prepared to address your issues. The above issues are best addressed with a physician or a psychiatrist, respectively.

3. **I am dedicated to my religion and very conservative when it comes to sex and orgasm. I am not sure if reading about sex is appropriate. Will I find this course helpful or offensive?**

This book is straight forward, direct talk about your body, emotions, lover and sexuality. I pull no punches. You will have a longer lasting partnership and a happier partner if you talk more about intimacy. You will experience a deeper connection and more fulfilling sex life. I bring sexuality out into the open where we can discuss our issues woman to woman and seek solutions by trying out specific exercises. If talking openly about sex is offensive to you, or talking about how to focus on sexual pleasure is against your beliefs, then I respect your position and this workbook is not for you.

Intimacy and sexuality are very personal matters. Not everyone is willing to open up and discuss or read about this subject. Choose this material wisely. I have no desire to be offensive or vulgar to anyone. My goal is to open you up to the beautiful, expressive being that you were born to be.

4. **Is this course for a specific age group?**

   The book is for adult women of sexual maturity throughout their lifetime. This manual is not for pre-sexually active teenage girls. I address all stages of sexuality, which are helpful for you to recognize. In your lifetime you will evolve and grow into your sexuality. There are challenges you will face during different phases. My hope is that this manual will sit in the night stand at your home and will be referred back to many times so that you can go back through the book and try new things.

5. **What if I am not comfortable doing some of the exercises in the course?**

   No one is here to watch over you and mandate that you complete each exercise. The exercises are all created for your benefit and only you will know if you did them. If they make you uncomfortable, then realize that this is an

Your Secret Chamber

opportunity for you to grow sexually. None of the exercises are painful, degrading, immoral, or harmful. Yes, you may be reluctant or embarrassed. That is a sign, to yourself, that you have areas where you are sexually limiting yourself. As you punch through these barriers, your orgasms will get better. If your body just responded to these words with excitement or fear and reservation, both are signs that your body wants to go further and enjoy the bonding experience of sex to fully envelope you. Why hold back from your own enjoyment? I can walk you through a process to open you up to the best intimacy you have ever enjoyed.

6. **Are you training in this field? How do you have the information to write this course?**
You could ask your doctor, mother or girlfriends about having orgasms, but you probably won't. And unless your doctor is a woman, he will not have experienced a female orgasm. There are people who are trained in women's anatomy and physiology, but the only way to be an expert in orgasms is to have them, lots of them, and understand through experience what makes them

better. I have also studied this subject, attended workshops, and coached women regarding intimacy and relationships for many years.

I've experienced some powerful intimate relationships. Some were deeply connected and others were powerful friendships. What I did was pay attention to what works for me. For eighteen years I have taught women how to have better orgasms. I will teach you how to pay attention to what works for you. Better orgasms will enriched your life, increased you happiness and bring pleasure to you and your lover. I share this information because I want you to enjoy your sexual experiences. It will help you and your partner to live better lives and grow closer together.

Chapter 1
The benefits of sex and orgasms

Honey I have a headache. Let's have sex.

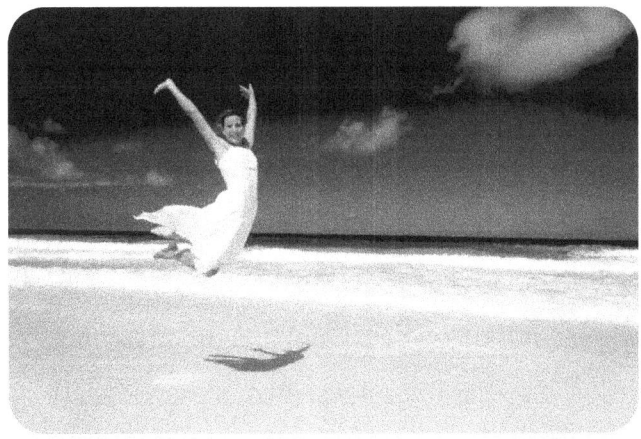

Stand up and speak. What do you long for? What do you want from your lover?

We are in the midst of great reform. No longer are you a silent partner in the bedroom. Road blocks,

Your Secret Chamber

beliefs and traditions have morphed to allow you to show your man all that you are born to be sexually and creatively. You are a caring, connecting, creative being that brings joy, love and life to the planet. You offer insight, intuition and softness, compassion and beauty. You are a mother and teacher to children, an empathetic ear and heart to your girlfriends and a lover and companion to a man. As acceptance of the feminine essence strengthens, you have more power to blossom and shine your sensual expression. Empowering yourself means accepting and expressing your inner beauty. You can take charge of your own sexuality and enjoy moving to higher and higher levels of pleasure.

During the Dark Ages, when feminine expression was restrained, sex became a taboo subject. We are still recovering from that programming.

Sex deserves much attention; especially orgasms! Intimacy is one of the best parts of life. Why don't more people make physical bonding a priority? The world would be a happier, less violent place if we did. Studies show that sex raises your mood, lowers your stress level, increases oxygen throughout the body, and is good for your heart. The benefits are numerous.

Your Secret Chamber

An overlooked advantage of sexual bonding is a man's ability to open you up to your authentic expression. You are a complex, emotional being who is often misunderstood. You can struggle to understand yourself. A loving partner, who truly sees you, can make you feel safe to open up to the radiant, enchanting, expressive creature that you are. Through lovemaking he can break down your walls so you can be the woman that you are capable of being. Sexual intercourse with a man accesses and stirs energy deep within you. When you trust and let down your walls, your man can penetrate to the depths of you to assist in bringing forth your inner essence. Together you two can find the sweet nectar within you. He can open doors to your inner soul that you won't find on your own. If you can see yourself through his loving eyes, suddenly you are empowered to express all that you can radiate.

Talking about intimacy greatly helps you be less inhibited so you can express your sensual self.

The more you read, talk about, hear about, or watch it on video, the more open minded you are about it. When you know that other people do something you haven't tried, then you may feel that you have permission to try that too. The more open-minded you are to great intimacy, the fewer walls you have that are hiding the real you.

Straight Talk

I want to start right out being very candid. I am going to speak to you direct and straight forward, the way you should talk to your man.

I have helped my friends and many women to understand and love their body so that they could let go into ecstasy. I can share the techniques. It's up to you to practice, but that's the fun part, because sex is your homework.

What you may not know is that there is much that you can do to enjoy outstanding orgasms. It's not all up to your man. I am not speaking about self-pleasure. I am talking about getting yourself ready to have great sex. If you are not ready, willing and able, your man can try as hard as he wants and still leave you unsatisfied. Your role is as important as his.

Do not leave your pleasure all up to your lover. Take control of your own sexual experience right now

Your Secret Chamber

by letting go of hang-ups, opening up to great sex, letting go and trusting, and learning what your body enjoys so you can communicate that to your partner. Leaving sex to chance guarantees you nothing. Just like most things in this world, it helps to educate yourself and practice. Sex takes practice and focus. It is not some passive activity you do just to please your partner. Sex is one of the best activities you can participate in for the health of your body and the health of your relationship. And yes, you must to participate actively.

Because this is a course in sexuality, you have some work to do while you read it. Well, that's partially true. There are activities you will be doing, but they won't feel like work, because they are all sex related. As a matter of fact, I call this a Sexercise Book instead of a course manual.

I want you to write about your experience; journal in this workbook about your progress so that you can continue to grow in this area. Writing has a different connection in the brain than talking and reading. Writing about your sexual experience will also take some of the mystery and secretiveness out of it. It will help you open up to more great experiences. Use a journal if you don't want to write in this book. Use this interactive Sexercise

Your Secret Chamber

book to its fullest by doing all of the sexercises. Each activity is designed to make you more comfortable with specific aspects of sex. It's a process and the actions guide your progression. You will do yourself a great service by doing all of the activities.

At the end of the book is a page for you to list all of the areas that you want to work on. When you come across a sexercise that you want more time practicing, list it on this last page along with the books page number for the sexercise. That way you can easily reference what you are working on, without thumbing through the book.

Included in this book are terms that are related to sex. Don't be surprised, or offended by these accurate terms. They must be in a Sexercise book in order to for me to communicate with you. Additionally I use these words to help you let go of hang-ups regarding sexuality. You want to be able to read and say the words cock and dick. Your man does not want you to <u>ever</u> refer to his member as a thingy, member or wee wee. He doesn't even like the word penis. Men have cocks or dicks, at least in their mind. And these are the words you should use. It is also a more exciting word for you to say than penis or member. So get used to the words cock

Your Secret Chamber

and dick. You will read them here many times. Soon sexy words will roll of your tongue as easily as the words great orgasm. I will also use words like anus, clit and oral sex. I will use the word penis many times, just between us girls. That doesn't mean you can use the word with your man.

Please know that these are the most accurate words to use. Reading all of these words will help loosen you up. If you are skittish about sex words and erotic words, then it is time for you to let go of hang-ups, blossom as a woman and open to the cosmic orgasms that are available to you. Spread your wings, physically, mentally and emotionally. The benefits are too good to pass up.

Your Secret Chamber

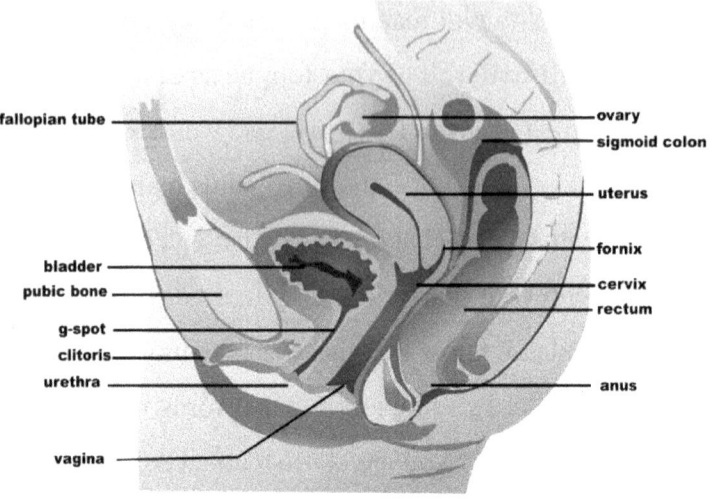

Review the drawing above. The area labeled as the fornix is the deepest place in your vagina and it is Your Secret Chamber. The word fornix is Latin for vault or arch. The deepest area of your vagina is a vault. Give your man the key and he will open you up to places you didn't know that you could go. I will teach you how to give him the keys to access to your vault for ultimate pleasure and opening up your authentic beauty.

The Benefits:

Men do not need to be told the benefits of love-making. Their needs and desires are proof enough to them of the importance of being intimate. Having excellent orgasms is a huge motivation for them. If you could have huge releasing orgasms each time you had intercourse, then you would want more sex too.

In addition to great pleasure, sex <u>IS</u> important for many other reasons. Here is a list of a few of the many benefits of having sex and orgasms.

1. Sex is great for your health.
2. Studies show that regular ejaculation in men is better for the prostate and lowers a man's risk of prostate cancer and that women who have more frequent orgasms live longer. *The Brain in Love* Daniel G Amen M.D.
3. Sex increases oxygen in the body.
4. Sex increases your heart rate and improves heart health.
5. Sex releases mood enhancing chemicals such as endorphins and oxytocin.
6. Regular sex improves loving relationships. Your love life is as important as your relationship. Many relationships dry up and fade away without regular sex. Sex creates a stronger, deeper bond for you and for him. Remember, sex

is a need for males, as much as feeling connected and loved is for you.

7. Sex can relieve a headache, stress and other tension related pain. An orgasm releases oxytocin which is a natural pain reliever. Next time you have pain, go to bed, with your partner. With a headache it is most affective to have sex when the headache is beginning and not after it has developed into something grand. Often sex is not an option when a headache initiates. If you are at dinner and a tension headache begins, you can't exactly grab your partner and run off to the bedroom. You could consider excusing yourself to the restroom and masturbate. The release of sexual tension often will alleviate other tension in the body. See tips on masturbation in the chapter called Let's Talk Orgasm. This technique may not work with headaches that are not caused by tension, such as migraines or dehydration headaches.

8. Sex boosts your immune system. Swapping saliva and bodily fluids boosts your body's immune response.

9. Sex increases circulation.

Your Secret Chamber

10. Sex burns two hundred calories in thirty minutes.
11. Sex builds a bonding connection with oxytocin.
12. Sex reduces pain through the release of oxytocin. (We sure like all that oxytocin does for us.)
13. Sex builds self-esteem and confidence by helping you feel desirable and sexier. Boosting self-esteem was one of 237 reasons why people have sex according to research conducted by University of Texas and published in Archives of Sexual Behavior.
14. Sex strengthens the pelvic floor muscle and helps with bladder control.
15. Sex helps you sleep better.
16. Sex creates relaxation.
17. Regular sex helps you produce more testosterone and sexual desire. That's right, you have testosterone too and it is what makes us want more sex. Use it or lose it.
18. Sex releases emotional aggression. It is much more than a physical release.
19. Sex keeps menstrual periods more regular.
20. Sex slows the aging process according to *Secrets of the Super young*, neurophysiologist David Weeks, M.D., of Scotland's Royal Edinburgh

Hospital, with regular sex shaving 4 to 7 years off your appearance.

21. Sex increases the pleasure you get out of life, physically, mentally and emotionally.
22. Sex creates healthier hair, skin, nails for both of you and healthier sperm for him.
23. Sex accesses deep parts of your authenticity through breaking down your walls, inhibitions and self-doubt. When a man can really see and open you, he can unlock the doors to your inner chambers to reveal your radiance.
24. Sex brings you to higher consciousness for achieving your goals. What are you searching for? Do you want money and fame or, fundamentally do you want peace, happiness and a fun life free of conflict? You are focusing on orgasms in this course, but the ultimate goal is a better life, more understanding, enlightenment and awakened consciousness. Orgasms can bring you to this place, ultimately. And the journey along the way is the best ride you can take.

Your Secret Chamber

With the exception of sexually transmitted diseases, there are no negative side effects of consenting sex. So have more sex. It is super good for you!!

Sexercise:

Write here which of these benefits you would like to gain from sex.

Sexercise: What are you not getting now that you want to gain? Better orgasms? More connection? Better sleep, circulation or happier mood? Feeling more open and authentic? Sex can give you all of these.

Write three benefits you want to gain here.

    1.
    2.
    3.

Sexercise: This first week have twice as much sex as you normally have with your partner. Notices the difference in how you feel. Write here about what you noticed.

Chapter 2

Hang-ups about Sex.

Get out of my way brain.

Let's admit it; women tend to have a lot of hang-ups about sex. Why? Good question. Most sexual hang-ups come from two places: parents trying to train you to be good a girl to keep you out of trouble, and societies' judgment about sex, including religions. I am not here to go head to head with any religious belief. Whatever your background or belief system, we can all agree that men and women have sex, sex is good for us, and sex is supposed to feel good. If we can all agree on these three things, then it doesn't matter what your background is or where your hang-ups come from. Your job is to overcome this programming that is holding you back from enjoying sex to its fullest potential. Doesn't that sound like a great plan?

Your Secret Chamber

My goal here is to help you get over any and all hesitations about healthy sexual activity. Again, my words are going to be blunt in this chapter. If you can read these words and not close the book, then you are that much closer to letting sexual hang-ups go and just enjoying all aspects of love making. Hold on to your seat and let go of being prudish.

Let's look at a few hang-ups:

1. **I find nudity and sex words offensive and distasteful.** Really? It's true that you might shy away from stories, jokes and discussions about sex. Perhaps you don't look at nude photos, would never go skinny dipping, and don't find looking at male parts super sexy or arousing. All of this is not helpful for opening up to sex. Becoming open to sexual pleasure requires embracing everything natural and healthy regarding sex and arousal. The only areas of sex to avoid are anything that is immoral, hurtful, or harmful. Talking about sex, using words like cock and clit, or even stronger words, and enjoying the beauty of the male body are all a part of embracing sexuality. It will make you feel more interested in sex.

Your Secret Chamber

2. **Good girls don't give or receive oral sex.** What? Where did this myth come from? Oral sex is an intimate, pleasurable, safe part of sex. If you think that it is unclean and smelly, then, let me be really blunt here; you are either in your brain listening to judgments, or you are not turned on, or you are not attracted to your lover. When you can get out of your head and into your body you will notice a few things about oral sex. First, it feels amazing to both the giver and receiver, if done correctly. Secondly, it is one of the most intimate and bonding activities you can do with a lover. Third it's a great way to build momentum towards a mind-blowing orgasm from penetration. This is such a vital part of good love making that I dedicated a chapter to it.

3. **Erotic stimulation is degrading and immoral.** Okay, I am not going to convince all people to change their minds on this one. But if you are on the fence, or curious, erotica can educate you and your partner, be very stimulating and spice up a stagnate love life. For occasional variety, some couples find it quite helpful. Men enjoy nudity, while women love steamy novels or romantic movies. Women have a better imagination and men love visual stimulation.

Your Secret Chamber

A university study in Australia determined that all men watch pornography and the average man began at the age of ten. I don't condone men watching regular pornography. Studies show that a lot of pornography can disengage men form the bonding aspect of sex. Men need visual stimulation of the female body, so you can provide that for him by showing him your sexy self, regardless of your size or weight. Nakedness is always sexy to your lover. Keep in mind that you can enjoy a sexy scene now and again, or a steamy novel, to get your mind engaged with the body. I wouldn't rule this one out when done tastefully and within healthy limits.

4. **I can't have my lover watch me masturbate or know that I have a vibrator.** I actually know women who hide their vibrator terrified that someone will find it. Give me a break. You should have a vibrator and know how to use it. Your lover should know how to use it on you. What a wonderful way to open you to your lover, to have him see you pleasure yourself or for him to pleasure you with a toy. Trust me, it is one of the BIGGEST turn-ons for a man. They love it. There may be an exception to this rule. Some men may feel threatened by a toy

that can please you. Just let him know that toys CANNOT do what his cock can do for you. The toy is only there to get you ready for the big daddy! Bring in the toys. New fun will be had by all. Your love life will enjoy new found pleasures.

5. **Fantasies mean that you are not connecting in a loving way and he is thinking of someone else.** Not true. I mention this in other parts of this book; when you fantasize together, it can strengthen your bond. Men desire variety in sex. It suits them well. Fantasies provide variety without changing partners. When the two of you are fantasizing together, you are the object of the fantasy; you as a nurse, you as a biker chic, or you as his doctor! Include fantasies for the ultimate enjoyment. Studies show that women's orgasms are more powerful when they fantasize.

6. **The lights need to be off so he doesn't see me naked.** If you only knew how helpful it is for your lover to see you, then you would never consider this. Men are visual creatures. I will say it many times. They like visual stimulation. They want to look at your breasts before they touch them. They want to watch their cock slide in and out of your body when they can. They want to see your beautiful face

Your Secret Chamber

smiling at them and the look in your eyes as they penetrate you. Keep the damn lights on! Soft lighting is flattering to your skin and shape. Use candles or dimmed lights. If you want your lover to open you up to the most authentic woman that you can be, he must see you, all of you!

7. **Being bound or held down is degrading.** If you have this hang-up, then you may not understand the benefits of being immobilized by your lover. The major goal for you during sex is to let go, open up, and allow yourself to be penetrated. That is the most common objective. Yes there are times when you may want to dominate. But surrendering and being taken allows for a level of letting go that your domination doesn't. For some of the best orgasms on the planet, you are submitting yourself to your partner and surrendering to his will. When you feel completely turned on and safe, surrendering thoughts will come to your mind, "You can have me. I'm yours, do anything you wish." Now, you can only feel that way when you trust your lover. If your lover is new to you, you might not get there for a while. But it's the best feeling when you let every inhibition go. You become ready for any penetration

and any touch. The reason he would hold your arms down, tie you up, or restrain you in some gentle way is to force surrendering a little. You allow your lover to tie you up and you are telling your mind and body, "I am surrendering now. Have me. Take me." It is not the same feeling as surrendering because you are so turned on and in full trust. It is more of an erotic feeling of being taken. There is a difference. Both are fun. I recommend being retrained on occasion. You can even include a blind fold and some spanking. While your movement is limited, practice letting go.

8. **Anal sex is disgusting.** Anal sex may not be for everyone. As you progress in the book you will learn that if you are having difficulty with orgasms, or you want to take your orgasms to higher levels, you desire one constant; more buttons pushed to reach that higher level of excitement. There are a limited number of buttons that you have available for sexual arousal, and I will talk about all the major ones. The clitoris wraps around the vagina and extends to the perineum and all the way to the anus. That is why many different types of stimulation feel so good. Anal stimulation is very arousing. It requires a little

preparation, which I will talk about later. But if you can get past this stigma, you are in for a rockin' good time. Anal orgasms can be pretty amazing for you and your man should love them as well. You can also just go for a little exterior anal stimulation. At the right moment it could send you over the edge of a wonderful waterfall into a sea of blissfulness. Don't rule this one out, even if you just take it a little ways, such as with fingers only. There is a plethora of nerve endings that will love you for it.

9. **I was sexually abused so I can't trust men or feel safe in bed.** This is a sensitive issue, and I feel for you. I can promise you this, many, many women were sexually abused; some statistics say one out of four women. Yet most of these women can enjoy sex. It is something that women can overcome. I know firsthand. There are many resources available to help you. Healing is possible and great orgasms are too.

Being open-minded in regards to sex allows you to have incredible orgasms that get better and better every year. You will want to get rid of these stigmas

Your Secret Chamber

so you can ignite energy in the bedroom and add a spark to your intimate bonding.

Sexercise:

Ask yourself if your current love making has become routine and lacks passion. If it does, which of these hang-ups are you holding on to? Or is there another hang up that I failed to mention here that you are holding on too? Write down all of your hang-ups.

Choose the first hang-up that you are willing to let go of today.
(Write here)

Practice doing the very thing that you were hung-up about.

Excellent work. Let's move on.

Your Secret Chamber

Chapter 3
Let Your Man Love You

> Your task is not to seek for Love,
> But merely to seek and find
> All the barriers within yourself
> That you have built against it.
>
> *Jelaluddin Rumi*

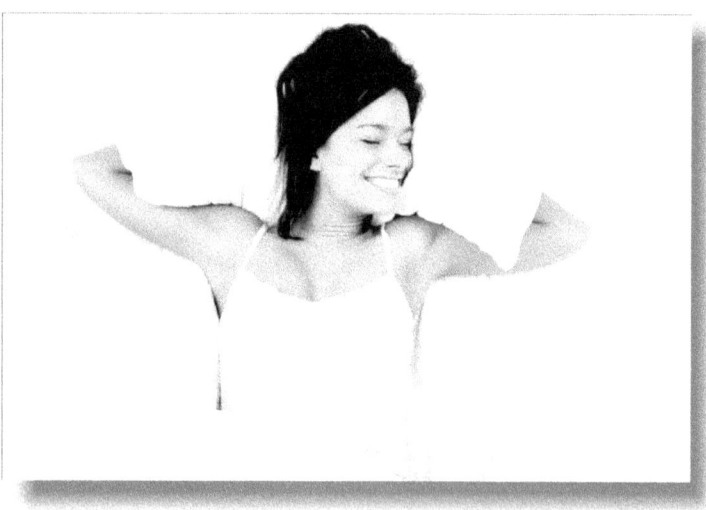

Learning to have great orgasms and giving a man full access to Your Secret Chamber requires removing the barriers you have built, like the walls you may have against love. Tension is a barricade to keep you distant from your lover. Tension is the wall that separates you from fully being loved.

Tension is most likely a part of your world. Maybe you worry. You fuss over people. You mend. You nurse. You feed. You give. You nourish and you become exhausted. A man will ask why you do this to yourself. The answer is -- because you are a woman. That's what women do.

Women experience more headaches than men because of the stress that they hold. Dr. Daniel G. Amen studied the difference in the brain waves patterns of men and women. When he asked men to relax their minds, eighty percent of their brain went inactive while twenty percent remained active. When he asked women to do the same thing, twenty percent of the brain went inactive while eighty percent remained active.

You may have a more difficult time relaxing than your man. You might hold upsetting news in your body by way of tension. Tension is the enemy of orgasm. Well, let me clarify that. Sexual tension is the fire in orgasm. Worry and anxiety is the enemy.

You can also experience depression or hormonal imbalances that can kill your libido. The causes are many and must be diagnosed individually. Food allergies, lack of nutrition and drug abuse can cause severe depression. Stress and tension can cause a hormone imbalance. Addressing these serious health issues is vital to enjoying a happy, healthy life.

Bad tension steals the energy from your body. When you are tense it is difficult for you to let go enough to have a very enjoyable orgasm. Stress is probably the number one reason why you can't have an orgasm on a particular night. It could be caused by emotional tension or negative thoughts, but it will stop you from having fun. Yes, it is possible to have a good orgasm while you are under pressure, provided that your brain does not get in your way. But you won't have a great orgasm, or the Big O, while you are tense. Big, bad orgasms require you to LET GO. You must release, relax, release, relax, breathe, be present, breathe, enjoy, release, open, breathe, relax, open, yes, yes, yes, that's the way!!

That is difficult to do with a headache, neck ache, stomach ache or whatever aches when you are holding tension. Let me emphasize a little psychology; tension is resistance. For example: you're tense because you're in a traffic jam. You are resisting what is going on in your world. You are tense because the babysitter left the house a disaster. You are resisting what is. If you can move through life accepting people, family and situations that you can't change, then you resist less and hold less tension. If you watch what is happening around you, and be a part of the experience instead of fighting it, then you are flowing.

I know, I know; easier said than done. As a woman, you may battle with this your whole life. It will take your lifetime, perhaps, to learn to accept what is and not allow it to cause you distress. Knowing that this is the goal, you can work towards less resistance.

Sexercise: Lie down and pay attention to your breath. Take several minutes to breathe deeply. Relax more with each breath. Now breathe as if everything in your world is perfect. Pretend that you are a woman who has come to terms with your past, your present, your body, your relationship, and all things in your world. All is well, perfect and how it should be. How does this woman breathe? It is slow, calm, intentional, relaxed and content. Now breathe this way for ten minutes or more. It will change your mood and fix things that you didn't know how to fix.

Your Secret Chamber

Your man can help you release tension by providing a safe, comfortable, non-judgmental environment for expressing yourself. In order for you to truly shine your feminine beauty, you must feel safe in expressing your unique, amazing, ever-changing, beautiful self without judgment.

Men sometimes think that they know what is best for you, but often their ideas limit who you are naturally. You will want to balance what your lover thinks is best for you with your own decisions. It is a process to be honed and practiced between couples.

Practice letting go. If you hold on to every little offense and some of the big ones, you will destroy your health, happiness and sex life completely. Learn to let it go. Release, relax, breathe, open, and achieve bliss! Life is short. Love is hard to find. Look for the good in your man and overlook his shortcomings!

There is another problem with male and female communication that is bigger than this book can fix, but I would like to touch on it. When you fell in love with your man you fell for a reason, other than simple magnetism. The man you fell in love with was your hero in some way, like a white knight on a great white horse. He was going to be a great father, or he was intelligent and stimulating to you, or he was going to provide for you, or he could have taught you things you didn't know. You fell in love because of something that man represented to you. Your man fell in love with you because of how you made him feel physically and emotionally.

The problem is that as you struggle to communicate and live life together, your man inevitably will disappoint you. It will happen. When he isn't the greatest father that you pictured, or he doesn't provide well for you, he makes a big mistake, or he doesn't do whatever thing that you thought you fell in love with, he falls off the white horse that you put him on. That is a big deal, because you may not know how to get him back on that horse so that you can feel good about him again. You may not even understand why you don't love him anymore.

So, before you let a little expectation ruin a loving relationship, see if you can't find another great reason to love the man you were attracted to instead of finding a new one. I guarantee that the next one has a very high chance of falling of the white horse too. You may not know how to keep him on the horse in your mind, so keep him on the horse in your heart by noticing

Your Secret Chamber

his great qualities and find a new reason to keep him on that horse. If you can't get him on the horse, you won't want to make love to him. I wish it were not true, but this is a fact that is helpful to know. Love your man even when he not your hero. Help him climb back on the horse.

Sexercise: Make the following commitments to yourself:

I will allow my partner to be a man. I will love him for who he is and appreciate his qualities.

_____
Signature

Sexercise: List your partner's qualities here. If you don't have a partner, list the qualities of a past partner.

Ways to Release Tension

Your Secret Chamber

1. **Take a hot bath**. Hot water will do wonders for you. Something about washing shifts the mood too, as if you are washing away the burdens of the day.
2. **Massage**. Of course! You desire to be touched in a non-sexual way. Being touched shifts your focus to your body, helps you relax, moves energy freely through your body and stimulates breathing.
3. **Lie down**. You can become overwhelmed. Sometimes you may not know when to say enough is enough. If you feel stressed, rest, clear your mind. Let everything go for a while.
4. **Write down your feelings**. Strangely enough studies show that talking to friends about our problems doesn't improve our mood. Yet, writing about them does. It has a different effect on the brain because it engages a different area. Next time you want to tell your girlfriends about a problem, consider writing about it. You will feel better.
5. **Watch a movie**. Distraction is good. Let it go for now.
6. **Have sex**. Sometimes tension in the body is sexual tension that you didn't realize.
7. **Meditate-Breathe**.

8. **Laughter** releases tension. Laugh hard and laugh often. Hold nothing back! Laughter is good exercise and fills you with oxygen. It releases good chemicals. When you laugh it exercises your vaginal muscles. Try laughing while you feel your vagina with your fingers. When a man is being funny and making you laugh, he is sending blood to your vagina and making it contract. Your vagina contracts along with your vocal cords. ☺
9. **Exercise**; it releases built-up energy.
10. **Scream, cry, make noise**, and let the frustration out in a sound. These activities increase circulation in the body and move energy. They also stimulate the vaginal walls to move and receive blood.
11. **Light some candles and listen to nice music**.
12. **Take a gentle walk**.
13. **Do a favorite activity** such as read a book, sew, or do a puzzle.

The point here is that there are many ways to bring the mind down and breathe in a relaxed state. If you can do this in the evening before going to bed, you will be much more open for sex and orgasm. If you are unable

Your Secret Chamber

to let go, and you try to control how things around you are going, it will get in the way of great orgasms.

One last note on tension: When you are tense, it is a bad time to speak with your partner. Please use one of the relaxation techniques before you converse with your partner on a sensitive subject. You might even want to write about it first. Hopefully your man can handle holding the garbage bag while you vomit your emotions at him. But how wonderful would it be for your relationship if he didn't see you vomiting often?

Sexercise: I will accept what I cannot change without allowing it to upset me and cause tension.

_____
Signature

Your Secret Chamber

Sexercise: List two examples of things that commonly upset you that you will accept as out of your control to change and that you will not allow to upset you.

1.

2.

Sexercise: I will make relaxing a priority in my life so that I can enjoy better orgasms.

_____

Signature

List the top five ways that you enjoy relaxing.

1.

2.

3.

4.

5.

Your Secret Chamber

Chapter 4

Let Your Man See You

If you do not feel self-conscious about your body, then chances are that you are not a woman. The most beautiful women feel self-conscious about something. As a woman you probably have a built in gene that makes you uncomfortable with your body. If you are lucky enough to have escaped this problem then hallelujah, there is hope for other women.

You may be self-conscious about your hair, toes, weight, face, eyes, complexion, voice, walk, clothes, breasts, or buttocks; you name it and you might feel that yours isn't good enough. Do you compare yourself to the prettiest woman that you can spot, noticing that you don't measure up? That's not good.

Get over yourself right now! Embrace your body and embrace your sensuality. There is perfection in the imperfections. You are unique and loveable. Commit to

Your Secret Chamber

begin to love yourself and appreciate the amazing woman that you are. Once you love and accept your body, you can enjoy everything sensual much more. Learn to relish and enjoy the amazing body that is taking you on this journey.

Start right now. How would you feel if right this moment a man was admiring your radiant beauty without any selfish intentions on his part? How do you feel when a man is noticing how amazing you are? Do you feel wonderful and beaming? You should. You are born to shine your essence.

Once you are able to let your man stare at your naked body and know every corner of it, then you are able to let him see your inner nakedness. Being comfortable with your body is being comfortable with yourself. If you want to open to your full potential, show your lover your body and then he will really see you.

Sexercise: Write down your best assets. Yes, you have them. Your best asset could be your smile, your hair, your voice, your eyes, your breasts or your ability to calm others or read poetry. Write your top five assets here:

1.
2.

Your Secret Chamber

3.

4.

5.

You have something sexy about yourself as well. Write the two sexiest things about your body:

My two sexiest assets are my_____ and my _____.

Excellent. You are beautiful. You are still going to maintain that beauty with good self-care. Not only will you pay attention to hygiene, such as going to the dentist and staying healthy, but you will maintain your hair, clothes, nails, skin and diet.

Remember that your man is a visual creature. Looking good for your man is as important as feeling sexy. Women are the flowers of the earth. Blossom for your man, and don't get too upset if he admires other flowers. That's like beating a dog for wagging his tail.

Sexercise:

Try all of these tips to looking and feeling sexy.

- Make your walk work for you. Be aware of your pelvis when you walk. Sway your hips and keep

Your Secret Chamber

your shoulders back. Walk like you are a tall, sexy model. It will make you feel much sexier. Men rate your sensuality based on your walk.

- Walk, sit and stand as if there is a man admiring your radiance with no selfish intent. He is just enjoying your beauty. Feel it all the time. It will help you feel sexy and, as a result, look sexier.
- Smile at others. Make eye contact. Show confidence. Your posture is the key. If you walk and stand like a confident woman, you will automatically feel more confident.
- Be aware of your pelvic muscles during the day. Squeeze them often. If you are able to build up some sexual arousal during the day, then breathe that energy up through your body. Pull that energy into your heart. Feel that arousal throughout your body.
- Open your heart by breathing in deeply and imagine that you are breathing the air in through your heart. As you expand your chest, imagine that you are expanding your heart as well, making it bigger and more receptive. An open heart will help you feel like you are more inviting to your lover.

Your Secret Chamber

- Get in touch with your feminine beauty that this masculine world depletes from us.
    - Dance like a fairy in the wind
    - Dress like a woman; wear girly, flowing clothes. Show off your curves.
    - Choose a woman that you think represents femininity well. Decide how you can emulate the feminine energy the same way she does.
- Be friendly while you embrace being a woman.
- Wear beautiful underwear. This helps tremendously. Each day when you dress you will feel more attractive with your pretty panties and bra hidden for later viewing.
- Spend time and money on your hair, nails, skin and lips. Maintenance is key. Look your best to feel your best.
- Love your body. Always focus your mind on your best assets. Do not look in the mirror and look straight at your flaws. Notice your assets and beauty.
- Exercise.
    - Each morning when you first get out of bed do fifty sit-ups. If you do that every day you will notice a firmer tummy in six months or less. If

you can manage to exercise thirty minutes each morning, it will do wonders for your fitness level and appearance.
  - Do your Kegels every day. Not only will your vagina be stronger, but so will your bladder muscles and pelvic floor muscles.
- Make a check mark next to every one of the above sexercises that you did.

Sexercise:

Write here areas that you <u>can</u> improve upon. I will to work on the following to feel sexier:

1.
2.
3.

Sexercise: Filling in the sentence of commitment.

I know that being sexual begins with feeling attractive. I commit to improving how I feel in these areas. I, _____, commit this _____ day to improve how I feel about my body by doing the following things;

Chapter 5
Learning to Blossom

Your Secret Chamber

Women and cats will do as they please, and men and dogs should relax and get used to the idea.
Robert A. Heinlein

Like flowers, the most delicious part of you is in the center of your bloom. That delicious center is your authentic self; your fears, dreams, challenges, ambitions, history, laughter, smile, and your unguarded eyes, heart and soul. To let go is to bloom, to open the flower, trusting that it is safe to reveal the center of your soul and to have faith that the one that you reveal it to will relish this gift and do all he can to protect its safe keeping. If your man never gets a glimpse of your center, he doesn't know how precious the flower is that he is protecting. You must let him see.

Just because you want him to see the center of your beautiful being, doesn't mean that you know how to reveal it. You must FEEL a certain way in order to open. The myth is that your man is responsible for how

Your Secret Chamber

you feel. It's true that your man can make you trust him, provide for you, protect you and pay attention to your response as he touches you or approaches you. But your man is not responsible for how you feel. You are! Right now you are taking charge of your own sexuality. Right now you can decide not to blame your inhibitions on your past. Right now you can begin a process that leads you to opening your heart so you can blossom and fully orgasm for your man. There is nothing your man will enjoy more than opening you up to your inner-beauty. Your bloom and pleasure is his reward.

      The secret is that your man can access doors to your inner soul and authentic expression that you struggle to unlock. Through his focus on your loveliness and by earning your trust, you give him the key to your secret doorways, the vault, where he can discover the incredible feminine radiance that you have waiting inside. The keys are in the deepest part of your vagina and throat and other sexual arousal areas that open you more fully to feminine luminescence.

Your Secret Chamber

> You are like a puzzle. A man enjoys the challenge of unlocking the riddle, turning all the right gadgets until he solves the mystery of you. On a deep level he knows that if he unravels you, a glorious reward awaits him.

To find the keys to your secret doorways he must solve the puzzle of how to bring you to orgasm. Perhaps you have an easy time with orgasm. Or maybe having an orgasm is not an easy task. Maybe you cannot have an orgasm anytime you want to. Perhaps the stars in the heavens must be lined up just so. Okay, not exactly, but if you are not feeling well, are injured, tense or emotionally hurt, the chances that you can relax enough to let go into pleasure are very small. When you are angry or hurt, you are often too distracted to cum. It helps significantly to be in a pleasant mood physically and emotionally.

Medical research shows that not all women have the same amount of nerve endings in the vaginal and clitoral area. Some women's nerve endings also extend further into the vagina than others. All women have nerve 'legs' that extend from the clitoris into the vagina and down to the anus. The women who have less sensitivity can do more intense activities to receive stimulation. I know of one woman who could not orgasm until she had her clit pierced. Now she reports that she orgasms every time. Women are not all made the same, and each have different ways to become aroused.

A man, however, could be in a mummy cast with many broken bones and he will still fantasize about his nurse making him cum.

For women pain is generally very distracting. Many things can sidetrack you from enjoying the pleasures of sex; kids in the house, company, someone being able to hear your moans, bills, something your lover said that hurt your feelings, or even something someone else said that hurt your feelings.

You are built to connect with another, on many levels. People are not designed to live alone, isolated from others; although some have proved it possible. Innate in our genetic makeup is the desire to bond and socialize. The more love, touch and connection that anyone has, the healthier they will be on many levels. Healthier people create a healthier planet. Sexual release also relieves anger and restlessness, allowing more peace. Some adults will never marry and some will never be in a committed relationship. Yet, the greatest intimacy and opening of their heart that they will enjoy will be with a sexual partner. Sex offers everyone many health benefits, with or without commitment.

We have many requirements that must be met in order for us to open up and let go into ecstasy. What does it mean to let go?

Five Basics to Bliss

There are five areas in which your needs must be met in order for you to open fully. These are not the exclusive responsibility of your partner. You have to meet him halfway. I will explain that in more detail below.

Please go through these five areas and rate yourself on a scale of one to ten in regards to your current partner. If you don't currently have a partner, rate yourself regarding a past lover.

The five areas are:
1. Trusting your partner
2. Feeling sensual, attractive and accepted
3. Feeling a connection

Your Secret Chamber

    4. Feeling cared for

    5. Self-care.

1. Trust:

<u>Trust is really number one</u>. I cannot emphasize this enough. If you want outstanding sex, you must trust your man. How can you show your most vulnerable secrets and inner most delicious place to your man if you cannot or do not trust? You won't do it. You are not built that way. You may have sex with a man you don't trust, but you won't open your vault and bloom.

    It's all about your vulnerability. Once a man knows every secret about you, then he could manipulate you, or take advantage. That is why you must trust him first in order to show him your vulnerability. Until then, your walls are up; like a tight bud.

    Trust includes honesty; two people being real with each other. Without honesty, trust cannot flourish.

    How do you know if you can trust your man? You have your ways of knowing. One way is through communicating what is important to you and what you like. If you tell a man that something is important to you, and your request is ignored, then you will feel that you cannot trust that man. For example, if you said that you hate to be tickled, and then you allow your lover to tie you up and he tickles you, then obviously you cannot trust this man with your heart. He won't protect what matters to you most.

If your lover says, "I will fix that oil leak for you," and then he doesn't ever do it, then you know that you are not important to him. This evaluation requires good communication. Before you decide that you can't trust this man, you might ask, "Is there a reason why you said you would fix my oil leak but you didn't do it?" There may be a legitimate reason.

However, if you have already opened your heart fully to a man who doesn't protect your best interest, then he can manipulate you into believing that there is no reason for you to expect him to help and protect you. That is simply not true of a loving relationship. If a man has no interest in helping and protecting your wellbeing, there is no reason to trust him.

Men feel a natural desire to help a woman they care about. Even when they're not in a committed relationship, and may only have a sexual connection with you, they can care about you and fix your car, help you move, be a date for a special event or have you over for dinner and a football game. These men can be trusted with your precious center nectar. You can open up your

Your Secret Chamber

inner beauty to them. They will provide help to you even though you aren't their girlfriend and they know that you never will be. These men can love you without commitment, and you can open your hearts and flower by being open to them. There are levels of love outside of the boundaries of a committed, monogamous relationship.

If you are feeling right now that trust is overrated and that there is no reason to be this vulnerable, then you are afraid to trust. Those thoughts are a manifestation of fears regarding giving your heart to another or fears about trusting others. Trust is an important aspect of a relationship. You can take baby steps towards trust until you are ready to jump all in.

In order to open to your lover fully, you must completely trust that he has no intention of harming you and that he has your best interest at heart. Think about your current lover, or a past lover. On a scale of one to ten, ten being complete trust without reservation, how much do you trust right now. Be honest with yourself if you want to make progress in this area.

1 2 3 4 5 6 7 8 9 10 Circle One

Sexercise: List here reasons why you hesitate to trust fully and ways that your lover could earn your trust.

Your Secret Chamber

Also look into your past and childhood. Are you projecting trust issues from your past onto your present lover? That is not fair. You want to evaluate your lover's protection of your heart based solely on his merits and not people from your past.

Reasons why I don't trust:

Ways he can earn my trust:

This workbook is not designed to fix emotional trauma and deep trust issues. I am making you acutely aware of the importance of trust. If this is a challenging issue for you, then now you know to explore this issue with experts so that you can learn to trust your partner and give him access to your inner radiance.

Sometimes a man may be doing everything he can to earn your trust and be willing to protect you fully, but you won't allow him because of things that happened before you met him. Until you trust him, know what your needs are and kindly and directly communicate those to your lover.

Your Secret Chamber

Sexercise: Tell your lover in a sweet, clear way what would make you feel safe in bed with him. Do not have this discussion halfway to the bedroom. Do not have this discussion when he is engaged in the garage on a project or watching TV. Ask him to set aside some time to speak with you when he is not busy. Men are single-focused. They cannot concentrate on two tasks simultaneously. Wait until you have his undivided attention. Then be honest and sincere. If he has no interest in the discussion, then you probably cannot trust him with your beautiful heart and won't be able to open to him fully.

2. **Feel sensual, attractive and accepted**

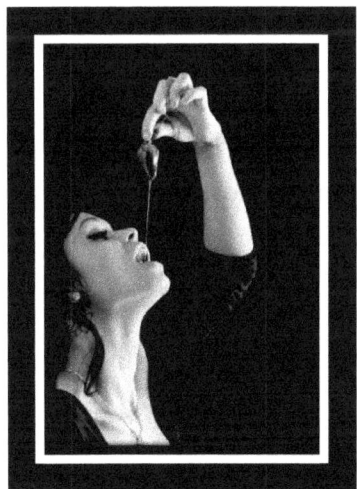

Your Secret Chamber

    Feeling sensual and attractive takes more work on your part than on your partner's. He can help you feel attractive by telling you that you are beautiful, but it is important that you feel good about yourself, even when your man is not stating how attractive you are. Your lover would not be with you if he did not find you attractive.

    Additionally, you want to be as authentic as possible so your man can see you. There is seeing that is physical which is your lover noticing your beauty. But there is a deeper level of seeing you, which is where he sees your mood on your face. He can see when you are tired. He knows the little subtle signals that you have and he knows when you are being honest or when something is bothering you. When you feel accepted you can be more open so that he can really see your true self. He can't know you on this level if you don't allow him to. It is really up to you first. Then he has to want to see you this deeply.

    You also must take the time to look and feel your best so you feel sexy and desirable. It helps to dress in ways that make you feel attractive and desirable. That does not mean slutty. When a man sees a woman in a bikini, or with her breasts hanging out, in his brain she

Your Secret Chamber

registers in the same place that everyday objects register. He sees her as an object and thinks, push the button, push in, pull out, and get pleasure. When he sees an appealing woman dressed femininely and her inner-beauty shining through, it registers in a different part of the brain associated with emotions, love, and attachment. Look beautiful, not slutty, if you want to attract a loving partner. For quick sex, you can do the opposite.

    Your posture, the way you walk, a sexy pair of underwear and even a flowing accessory can make you feel beautiful. Feeling attractive is an important component to building arousal and enjoying sex. There are many books, websites and seminars that can help if you feel like you want extra help in this area.

    One more important element is acceptance. You want your man to relish in the fact that you are a woman. You flow. You express. You shine and you're unique. Often men are quick to judge women. Men come from a different perspective and may judge a woman as irrational, too sensual in public, or as having poor judgment. If you feel reluctant to be yourself, or to say what you think, or express who you are fully, you will not be able to blossom for your man. He must accept you without harsh criticism, or he will not get to experience the fullness of your beauty.

Your man has a goal of opening you up so he can see you blossom. He knows the value of discovering your delicious, secret center. But he also has other motivations that are a part of his genetic makeup. If you want to interact in a sexual nature with men, you must accept that sex is a need for males, as much as feeling connected and loved is for women.

If their desires or your desires are not met, then the relationship suffers. You and your partner will benefit by giving to each other in order to receive what you each want. Who is going to give first? If you each withhold, waiting to get what you want, everyone suffers. You are a giver by nature. It's not too late to begin enjoying your orgasms so much that you want to give your partner regular lovemaking. Soon he will be happy to please you in order to keep receiving what he must have.

If you achieve mind blowing orgasms every time you have intercourse, you will decide to have it more often. For men, orgasm is an easier task. With practice, it can be easy for you also. Your relationship with your lover or husband will improve significantly if you are

Your Secret Chamber

having outstanding orgasms. Not only will you want more sex, but you both will have a much better experience.

Think of it this way. You know that men need food and sex right? Allowing your partner to penetrate you to satisfy his needs while you are not pleasured is just like serving your partner cold mashed potatoes and gravy or cold clam chowder for dinner. True, he won't starve because he still gets the calories, but the enjoyment would be much improved if the food where hot!! Sex for him will be so much better if you are hot!! Hot for him, hot looking, and hot about sex. Serve his gravy hot and be the flavor that spices up his world. He will love you more deeply for it.

Another aspect of men that you want to accept is that men want variety. They desire sexual stimulation, such as seeing you naked or watching a sexy movie. Sex is on their mind throughout the day, but they don't have the visual imagination that women do. That is why they seek visual stimulation. Men in committed relationships entertain themselves with magazines, movies and internet options regarding sex. You may find this very upsetting. But it is not an unusual activity to occupy their minds that is constantly returning to thoughts about sex. Studies show that single men view porn twice as often as men in relationship view it.

The best thing that you can do to keep his thoughts about you, is to give him lots of variety and lots of visual stimulation. Routine sex becomes boring for your man. There are many ways you can spice things up.

Sexercise: Choose three of the following activities to create variety with my lover:

- Dress sexy
- Change positions
- Use toys
- Enjoy erotica together
- Fantasize together
- Try something new
- Play a sexy character, then jump out of bed and leave the room after sex to change up the routine. Keep it shallow and he will beg for cuddling next time.
- Make a sex date, where the whole evening is about you looking hot and you enjoy steamy sex without any other agenda.

Your Secret Chamber

- There are so many ideas that you could do. He won't want to do all of the work regarding variety. He will love it if you will come up with some ideas. Be creative to keep his interest and you will make him want to come back for more.

Sexercise: Write here about the three you chose and how that made a difference.

How attractive and desirable do you feel?

1 2 3 4 5 6 7 8 9 10

Sexercise: Make your partner aware of how it feels to you to know that he appreciates your beauty. He may not know that a huge component for you opening up to him comes from him finding you desirable. You are a beautiful being. When he notices this, you will show him more of your beauty. He responds by noticing you further, which causes you to open wider. He reacts by noticing how open and lovely you are and so you show him some of your inner beauty. He enjoys it so you allow him to see your nakedness. He loves looking at your body and this allows you to show him your inner nakedness. He relishes it and protects that with his life.

3. Feeling connected to your partner

In order for you to open your heart, body and soul to a man, you must feel a connection with him. Connections can happen in seconds or it may take a while, or it might not happen between two people. The reason you want to go to dinner with a man is to try to connect. If he talks only about himself, doesn't listen well and isn't present, you have no interest in going further. You will feel most connected to a man when he is fully present with you. Have you experienced being fully present with another person? If you have then you will understand what it means. All of the words in the world could not adequately describe the feeling. There are endless levels of feeling connected. I don't believe that you will ever achieve the highest point of connection; it can grow infinitely.

However, the more connected you feel with your partner, the more open you can be. Open means everything, including throat, vagina and heart. You cannot allow your partner to comfortably penetrate you to the deepest parts of your vagina unless you are fully open.

Your Secret Chamber

Often you will want to talk before lovemaking. This is so that you can accomplish two things; to get your distracting thoughts or hurt feelings dealt with so you can relax and get in the mood, and to connect with your lover. Both of these are important. If something is on your mind, and you can't set it aside, then it stays in your brain while you're naked. Then you can't enjoy yourself. Keep in mind that it is better if you can talk about the distractions long before it's time to make love. Although you will feel more connected with your partner when talking in bed, he may feel distracted. Suddenly you feel better and ready to go and he wants to go watch football and tune out after the emotionally draining conversation. The best thing that you can do is to address your emotions as they arise, in the moment, and not as you are walking into the bedroom with your lover.

You may have a difficult time communicating when you feel hurt. Words do not flow to you and you don't know how to explain your feelings. Days later you might be able to articulate why something that your lover said hurt your feelings. The problem is that days later he has forgotten the entire situation. He has no frame of reference. His thought will be, "Why are you bringing this up now. That was ages ago." To a man three days ago may as well have been three years ago. Now you are blaming him for things he did in the past. That makes him feel ambushed and frustrated. In his mind he is trapped because he can't fix the past or even remember the details.

What a man wants is to know right when he hurts your feelings so he can fix it right then. Men are solution oriented. "How can I fix this?" So when you can't find the words, make a sound, "Ohhh." and a facial expression. Once your lover knows that this is how you explain a hurt feeling or even anger, then he can tune in and ask what occurred to hurt your feelings. You should explain ahead of time to him that you usually won't be able to verbalize to him why your feelings are hurt right then. But what you want in that moment is reassurance. He could put his arm around you and explain to you that he didn't intend to hurt you. If you two are on the phone he could say he is sorry for the unintentional hurtful words. Ninety-five percent of the time your man has no intention of hurting your feelings when he does it. But you are a sensitive creature because you are female. He wouldn't love you the same if you were insensitive.

How connected do you feel to your partner?

Your Secret Chamber

1 2 3 4 5 6 7 8 9 10

Connecting with your partner takes practice. You may have so many distracting and self-conscious thoughts that you rarely stay fully present and engaged during lovemaking. Yet staying present, and fully aware of all of your sensations, will allow you to go to the next level of pleasure. This component is so essential that the next chapter is dedicated to the subject of being present.

Your Secret Chamber

Sexercise: Do all of the following:

1. Set aside some time to have a deep conversation with your lover. Take turns taking about things that will help you feel connected with each other. Be good listeners. Have eye contact and make that connection. Feel the bond strengthening between you.
a. Write about what you notice from this conversation.
2. Take five to ten minutes to stare in your partner's eyes while touching and caressing each other's hands. Stay present and connected with each other. See if you can dance your hands in a rhythm that you both can follow and anticipate while looking only into each other's eyes. Feel the connection.
3. While making love, take as much time as you can to stare into each other's eyes. Communicate your pleasure with your eyes as well as your body. With your eyes, read each other's wants, desires and pleasure by being present. When you feel you are losing the connection, say something to your partner; "Hi. There you are. I feel you again. Thanks for being right here with me." You will automatically notice when the connection is lost.

Your Secret Chamber

Feeling Cared for

You are caring and giving, but you also have an innate desire to feel cared for. This may scare you if you choose to be intimate without a committed relationship because you want your independence. You might be trying to make sure that your partner does not do things for you so that you don't feel obligated to him. If you fit into this category, then I have good news. You don't have to be a wife, or be financially supported by a man to feel cared for. It's not necessary to have your man take you to fancy restaurants or buying you fancy clothes. There and many was to be cared for.

However, it's not true if you say, "I only want my lover for sex. I don't want anything else from him." That's not exactly right. You don't need much from your lover to have sex and orgasm. But without feeling cared for, you could have nearly that same level of orgasm by yourself. That's the bad news. To have better, deeper, richer, more fulfilling sex you must feel cared for. This is natural to us and perhaps goes back to the days when women were more dependent on men and possibly often repulsed by them. Think of the caveman days; Men were uncivilized, hunters of wild game, warriors, and poor communicators. They were smelly, hairy and less gentle. (Please excuse my generalization to make a point) Yet men provided for the women and protected them. This was how they cared for the women. Their care and assistance softened the women so that they could be open to receive a smelly, hairy man. If a man were to grab you for sex, without the show of genuine affection or caring for you, you would resist, be closed and unable to enjoy him.

Regardless of how independent you are, you want to be appreciated and cared for by your man before you can go 'To the Moon and Back' with him.

In a loving relationship you like to feel that a man thinks about your future together. In a sexual relationship, with or without love involved, you want to feel safe and significant or special. Innate in you is a desire to feel provided for, either financially, or by a man being helpful, such as teaching you things you can't do on your own. On a primal, subconscious level, you like a man to provide something for you in exchange for sex and your nurturing devotion. A balanced exchange allows you to give the most you can. But you will do this unconsciously. It is not as if you are thinking, "What's in it for me?"

Your Secret Chamber

Of course sometimes you may be in a period of your live where you only want a sexual relationship. At these times you still have other desires. You want to know that you are safe, that there is a level of respect and caring, even if it is just for the night. You also love to feel attractive. In these purely sexual relationships you are getting far more than just sex. You are receiving all of the above, plus human intimacy, interaction, connection and health benefits.

If you are in a long-term relationship that has lost some of its luster, then you must get proactive today to inform your partner what makes you desire more intimacy. If your partner is still with you, most likely he cares for you deeply. Men generally love deeply and stay with the women they adore. They often, however, forget to show that devotion. Keep in mind that men show how they care in different ways. Here are a few examples; Chopping the wood, hunting for food, going to work, cooking, saying that you look nice, saying "Thank you," for dinner, giving you a gift or compliment, saying, "I appreciate you," listening to you, making you something, being compassionate when you feel ill, cleaning the car, washing the dishes, mowing the yard, doing something to make you happy.

Your Secret Chamber

Sexercise: Write down here five ways in which your partner is showing that he cares for you.

    1.

    2.

    3.

    4.

    5.

On a scale of one to ten, how cared for and appreciated do you feel?

1 2 3 4 5 6 7 8 9 10

Sexercise: Write down additional ways that you desire him to show his appreciation for you.

    1.

    2.

    3.

    4. **Self-care; making time for pleasure.**

This is more important than you may realize. You are nurturing and giving. Often that leaves no time for you. You've heard it before; you must feed your own

Your Secret Chamber

reserves or you will run out of energy to give. One of the absolute most important things that you can do for yourself is allow time for pleasure and indulgences. I am not talking about a half-gallon of ice cream. I am taking about what you are born for; gratification. You must allow all kinds of healthy sensation into your life if you want mind blowing orgasms. Below is a simple list to give you some ideas of what are basic pleasures that help you experience what you are born to enjoy. Your man does not desire these things the way you do because he is built for a different experience. You are designed for textile bliss.

    a. A hot bath
    b. A soft robe
    c. Perfumed body lotion
    d. A scented candle
    e. Flowers
    f. Chocolate
    g. A pretty journal
    h. A gift basket
    i. A clean baby
    j. A soft kitten
    k. Lying in the sun
    l. A walk on the beach

Your Secret Chamber

- m. A hike in the mountains
- n. A long massage
- o. Fresh baked cookies
- p. *Better than Sex* chocolate cake
- q. Reading a romantic novel
- r. Having tea with girl friends
- s. Taking the kids to the zoo
- t. Taking an afternoon nap
- u. Pretty clothes
- v. Soft anything
- w. Jewelry
- x. Laughter
- y. Hugs
- z. Being spoiled

Do you see it? Can you tell that you are built to experience decadence? Indulgence and gratification are preludes to orgasm. If you are lacking basic joys of being a woman, then having orgasm will be more challenging and limited.

Sexercise: List here all of the indulgences you experience on a weekly basis.

Your Secret Chamber

Sexercise: Write the ones you will add to your regular experience.

On a scale of one to ten, how much enjoyment do you allow yourself for sensual bliss?
1 2 3 4 5 6 7 8 9 10

The Magic of 10-10-10-10-10

Sexercise: Look at your ratings above. Add up your total score from each of the five areas. Write your current score here in pencil (It will change over time)_____/out of fifty. Achieving five perfect tens is unlikely to happen often. It's something to strive for. The higher score that you get on these five scales will directly affect how powerful your orgasms are.

These five areas are not all that it takes to open yourself to your lover. But having these five things met allows for more fulfilling orgasms. You can have good sex and good orgasms without these basics being met, but it is less fulfilling and it will be difficult to reach your pinnacle of pleasure until the numbers on these scales get high.

Your Secret Chamber

Chapter 6
Being Present

Get out of your head and connect with your partner

> *The subject tonight is Love*
> *And for tomorrow night as well,*
> *As a matter of fact*
> *I know of no better topic*
> *For us to discuss*
> *Until we all*
> *Die!*
>
> ~ Hafiz

Your heart, senses and emotions are satellites; senders and receivers of a constant flow of information. When you observe life with focus, as it occurs, then you are present. When you are remembering past events or imagining the future, you are distracted from the present moment.

When you are present with your body, you make strong connections between body and brain. Your life is built around the different connections you have established between your body and brain. If you have established any negative relationships, then they will remain until you remove them intentionally. If you have negative connections between mind and body in regards to sexuality, it could stop you from having powerful orgasms. One way to heal these negative attachments is to be fully present with your body and listen to what it wants.

As you become more able to connect mind and body, you can establish acute awareness of what feels good to you sexually. You can pay attention during sex and notice what you like and what caused you to get aroused and enjoy a certain kind of orgasm. You can journal about it and work on recreating orgasms that you really enjoy.

Being present is more than just self-awareness. You also want to be aware of your partner. Being aware of your partner in an acutely-present way creates a strong field, building a great movement of energy.

I like using the lightning cloud for an analogy to explain this energy. Clouds builds up an electric charge as particles rub and bump against each other while they rise or fall within the cloud. Isn't that sexy? As particles bump together, they create a negative or positive charge. Oppositely charged particles create an electric field that builds up electricity. If the charge builds enough, an explosion must happen to diffuse the charge. It sounds remarkably similar to sex. The result in a cloud is usually an explosion of heat that you see as lightning and hear as thunder. Did you ever hear the phrase when you were a kid in a lightning storm that the gods where making love?

A similar thing happens then two people rub together. Friction causes heat and a powerful electric charge. But there is more. In a cloud the particles loose an electron and the air becomes ionized. That means that the particles in the air are electrically charged and they attract the oppositely charged particles creating a stored energy field between the negative and positive particles. Now, instead of rubbing against one another, they are paired. This also sounds sexy. If you could use your imagination you could say that they are no longer single, but two particles have become one field of energy.

Becoming one is something you want in love making, creating the friction and polar opposite attractions to merge your two energies. It is a beautiful feeling, yet perhaps it is not the whole story. There may be more than you can achieve than merging energies. Below Rumi tells us about love and oneness. Love has more to offer you than you may understand. Is it the soul's light that you pine for?

The Taste of Morning

Time's knife
slides from the sheath,
as a fish
from where it swims.

Being closer and closer
is the desire of the body.

Don't wish for union!

There's a closeness
beyond that.

Why would God

want a second God?

Fall in love
in such a way
that it frees you
from any connecting.

Love is the soul's light,
the taste of morning,
no me,
no we,
no claim of being.

These words
are the smoke
the fire gives off
as it absolves its defects,
as eyes in silence,
tears, face.

Love cannot be said

Rumi

      There is more to love than becoming one physically. In love making you can reach the soul's light, or an enlightened state. If you are present with your body and direct your sexual energy throughout it,

Your Secret Chamber

you can have an orgasm that takes us to new levels beyond merging energy.

I can give you many exercises for being present. Truly it is something that you must practice throughout your lifetime. This list is small and does not encompass all of the ways in which you can focus the mind on the present moment. So continue to seek ways to learn this empowering skill. Read books, go to workshops or learn deep meditation. It will not only help you with sex, but it will bring you to new states of enlightenment and improve your life as you journey along.

Sexercises:

1. Spend ten minutes staring into your partner's eyes. Notice what you feel. Ask him to notice you, to feel you. Is he opening up his soul to you, or are there walls he has placed to hide his inner world from you? Are you connecting? Pay attention to what you feel. Ask your partner to notice how you look to him. As he notices your beauty, you will open up to him more. Notice how his eyes make you feel.
2. During the day, while you are waiting in traffic or at the post office, be aware of your pelvic

region. Feel it. Do some Kegel exercises, notice the sensations. Pull that energy up through the body with your breath and intention. Do your Kegels by contracting your vaginal muscles, then the entire pelvic floor. Squeeze them all tighter and tighter until you can't squeeze them anymore. Then very slowly, release the contracting until your muscles have all relaxed. Do this ten times.

3. Practice opening your heart with breath and intention. Do this by breathing in deeply and imagining that you are breathing in through your heart.

4. Close your eyes and practice feeling your body. Tune out the world and listen to the rhythm of your body and head. You may be able to hear sounds from your body such as your heart beat. Check in and feel your body's sensations. Do you have tension anywhere? Do you feel any pain? How is your breathing? Is it deep or shallow? Notice every part of your body. Be present with your physical essence.

5. While your partner stimulates you, close your eyes and pay attention to exactly how it feels to

Your Secret Chamber

you. What sensations are spreading through your body? Now open your eyes and look into your partner's eyes as he stimulates you. Connect with your eyes and your bodies.

6. Learn more about how to become more present through mediation classes, videos or courses. Being present will change your world. Practice meditation and many doors of understanding will open for you.

Sexercise: Write down your experience with doing two of the sexercises regarding being present.

Sexercise: List any new ways that you will practice being present.

Your Secret Chamber

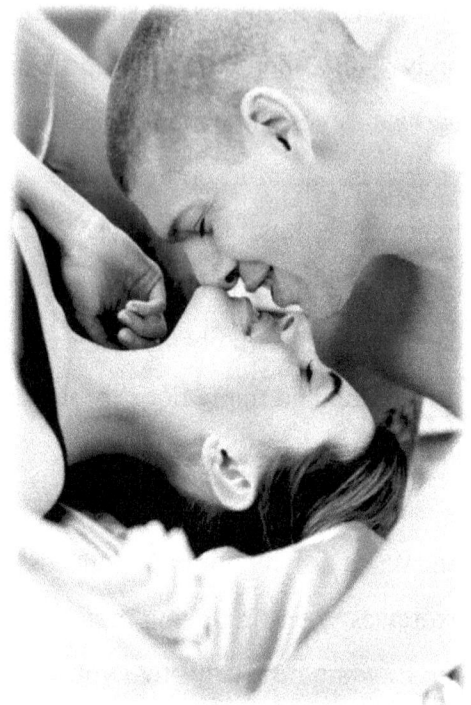

Sexercises: Complete all of the following this week.

Practice being present with your partner:

1. Ask your partner to do the following sexercises with you. Spend time kissing each other where you each concentrate on the kiss. Be acutely aware of your lips and tongue and your partner's response. Open your eyes and look at each other as you kiss. Pay attention to how your body responds as you kiss. Don't move on to other touching until you are both

Your Secret Chamber

very present with the kissing. Communicate with your partner when you feel him being present.

2. Take turns touching each other and watching the other respond to your touch. Focus on the other person's face and muscle movements. Without talking, see if you can both discover what each other likes best. Then share openly about the experience.

3. Take turns telling your partner something that you feel or an incident that happened to you. Do not use this time to share something difficult between you. Just share something personal. The listening partner just listens without speaking and notices the expressions and feeling of the one speaking. Then change who is speaking and who is listening silently. When each person has had a turn to speak, hold each other and just feel each other's heart beat and body language.

Chapter 7
Arousal is the Key to Pleasure

If you are proficient at having orgasms, then you are likely to be experienced at becoming aroused. The following information includes ideas to help you build up your sexual arousal so you can hit a higher climax. The most important thing to understand about orgasms is <u>that the more aroused you are, the higher your climax can be</u>. Orgasms are a release of energy. The more you release, the greater your pleasure.

Increasing your stimulation level is best done by stimulating more than one area. The more areas that are stimulated, the better that your orgasm will be, the better your relaxation afterwards, the more oxytocin that will be released, and the better your mood and health will be. Additionally, the more pleasure that you receive from lovemaking, the more sex you will want to have. The more sex you have, the better your overall health, vitality and appearance. There are so many benefits to

Your Secret Chamber

heightening your excitement, and that is why I will mention all of the many ways to become stimulated. Please don't take offense if you are not interested in one or more of these ways. You don't have to do them all. Just consider trying something new so that you can increase your sexual tension and therefore your pleasure, release, mood and health benefits.

We have already addressed many of the essential elements necessary to having a great orgasm. We talked about:

- being relaxed
- letting go of stress,
- letting worries go so you can fully participate
- feeling sexy and sensual
- being present and how to practice that
- sexual attraction and the value it brings to your excitement
- trusting your partner
- appreciating your body and knowing what your body likes
- communicating what you want to your lover
- feeling connected and cared for

- surrounding yourself with sensations and gratification

All of these things get you ready to enjoy the experience. If it sounds complex, that's because it really is. You are complex. Many times you won't even understand yourself. How can your lover understand you? If one of the above is out of balance, then you could have a difficult time reaching climax.

Once the above are in order, then comes the physical involvement. It is important for you to be physically active during sex. I have heard men complain about women who "just lie there". They don't move their hips or make a sound. If you are not moving or making a sound then you are probably not having a good time, because it's nearly impossible to hold still when you are building to orgasm or having one.

And vica versa, moving and making sounds make you feel more excited, even if you are not doing it automatically. Have you heard that if you smile it will put you in a better mood? Well it works. Your smile muscles are wired in your brain to trigger a feeling. Smiling is good for your mood. Likewise moaning and moving your hips is good for your sexual mood. Making

Your Secret Chamber

the same noises that you would during orgasm stimulate the vaginal walls, making you more aroused.

If you are not in the mood, there are <u>many</u> things that you can do to get yourself there. Participating in sex is an important element.

If you believe that you are less sensitive or have a hidden clit, then you can work harder than most at stimulation or look into more intense ways to receive stimulation, such as piercing, using ice, heat or firm vibration directly on the clitoris.

Even if you consider yourself a very sexual woman, there may be times that you are not in the mood for sex. Now that you know the huge benefits from sex, you have motivation to spend time to get yourself in the mood. Not being in the mood is not an adequate reason to skip sex. You know that your stress level will go down, your heart rate will benefit, your body will relax and it will build an ongoing bond with your partner. Those are all great reasons to jump out of your head and into your sexy body and have some fun. The best motivation you can have comes from having great orgasms.

Your Secret Chamber

Here is a list of many of the things that you can do to stimulate your mood and build arousal.

First the prep work, before you are with your man.

- **Make a list** of everything that you would do to prepare for a first date with a guy that you liked. Would you trim up your pubic hair, paint your toes, and fuss with your hair for an hour? You can do all of those things for your partner to spice things up. Write down here what you would do to impress a new hot guy.

- **Be sensual during the day and flirt.** Dress feminine, think about sex and what turns you on as you go about your day, flirt and be coy with your partner. Text him what you would like to do with him tonight, or invite him for a quickie at lunch. Tell him that you are not wearing panties, or let him know that you can see his cock in your thoughts right now. Be coy and cleaver. Tease him a little. He wants you. Increase that sexual tension.

Your Secret Chamber

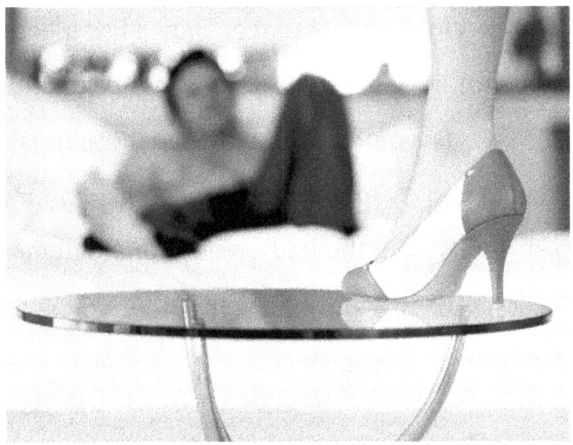

- **Dress up!! Get your grove on girl!** Put on some lingerie. Wear a skirt without panties. Wear your sexiest underclothes. Put a fake tattoo on your body so he can find it. Glitter your skin, put on a wig, dress like Lady Gaga, don your high heels, wear sexy boots with your negligee, wear a seductive mask, play a character of a powerful, seductive woman. You are beautiful and desirable. OWN IT!! LET HIM KNOW IT!! Seduce him. He craves variation in your love making.
- **Walk the talk.** A sexy walk includes moving your hips side to side with your shoulders back. Do you have a sexy walk? Confidence is the key. Own it girl. It's all yours to show off.

- **Dance your sexy essence.** Dance has a benefit you may not have thought of; moving to sexy music moves your mojo around. Move those hips, stir your sexual energy up, and express your feminine sensuality. Get the body ready for excitement.
- **Use a vibrator on yourself** before you see him to get a quick boost.

Things that <u>you</u> can do with your partner to get yourself in the mood:

- **Chemistry.** Steamy hot chemistry is enough to create some exciting explosions all on its own. Chemical attraction is a powerful force that we don't fully comprehend. It's beautiful when two people have chemistry for each other. In some relationships one person feels more physical attraction than the other. You can take advantage of the chemistry by focusing on it. You will often get the chemistry triggers from looking into his eyes, smelling him with a deep breath, looking at the parts of his body that most turn you on, tasting his saliva from kissing, tasting his skin, feeling his touch, and hearing his

Your Secret Chamber

voice. Use chemistry to your advantage to get aroused.

- **Touch him.** If you are not particularly excited, then begin touching your partner and having him caress you. Talk about parts of his body that you enjoy. Touch your favorite spots on him. Take some time for this. No hurry. Enjoy each other's body. Touch all of the spots on him that you find arousing. Keep in mind that the whole time you are close, and even before you entered the bedroom, your man is thinking, "When is she going to touch my cock." It is true. That is what they want to know. So touch it, as soon as you are ready. The sooner the better for him, but you don't want him to be ready to explode before you.

- **Strip show.** Taking your clothes off slowly with some music can set the mood for both of you. When you see how interested he is in you and how captivated he is by you, you will be aroused by all of that attention. When a man that you feel safe with focuses his attention on you, you will automatically open up more. Take it off slowly. Tease him. Show off your breasts and your good parts. Brush his legs with your bare ass. Let your hair slide across his face and shoulder. Get close, then back up. Do what comes natural. You are a woman!! Make him want you. A fun twist on this is to ask him to undress you. Give him playful encouragement. Brush his skin and put your hand down his pants. But allow him to remove all of your clothes, without your help.

- **Kiss his body,** anywhere you like. Enjoy his taste and smell.
- **Kiss his cock/dick.** Just a few kisses, licks and close touches can do wonders for both of you.
- **Give him a blow job.** I will talk more about this in a separate chapter, but done well, this can be extremely arousing to you. If you do it for yourself and just enjoy how wonderful his cock feels to your lips, tongue and mouth, you can even have an orgasm from giving head.
- **Make sounds like you are having an orgasm**. The throat is so connected to the vagina, and the brain is so involved in your orgasms, that when you make the sounds of a great orgasm, you are releasing sexual tension and bringing on an orgasm. So open your throat with sounds, don't keep it tight and high

Your Secret Chamber

pitched, and let out the most animalistic moan of pleasure that you can possibly muster. Don't let your man think that you are all done though. You are just getting started and you are just letting the juices flow!

- Once he has penetrated you, **move your hips**, even if it is not automatic. This will get you excited.
- **Squeeze your vaginal muscles**. These muscles contract during orgasm. If you contract them intentionally, you will bring yourself closer to orgasm. This will stimulate you and him. Often his penis will response by bulging from excitement, which will stimulate you as well. Practice squeezing the vagina muscles often during the day. Keep that muscle strong and healthy!!
- **Squeeze your entire pelvic floor**. These muscles also naturally contract during orgasm. This is so important to build excitement, especially prior to orgasm. When you squeeze your vaginal muscles and pelvic floor muscles, it can take you much more quickly into orgasm. When you want to delay an orgasm that is building, then relax all of your pelvic floor muscles and draw the pleasure up through your

body by breathing deep and spreading the feelings through your whole body. I will talk extensively about this in the chapter, *Meet you at the Top.*

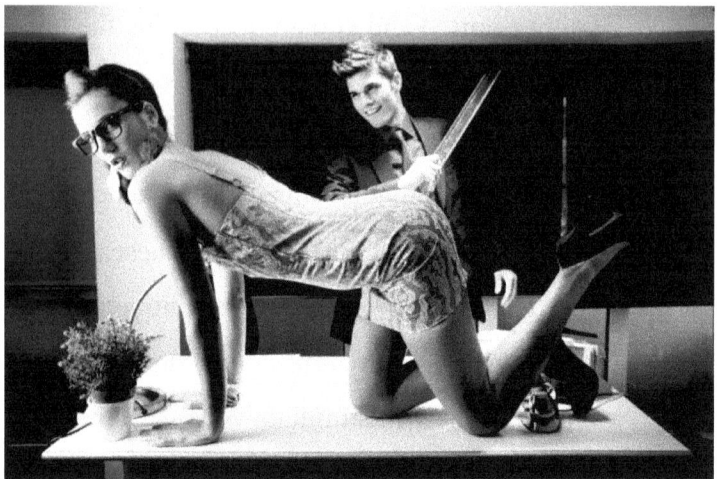

- **Fantasize.** Fantasies can be so vivid and strong that both men and women can have an orgasm from fantasy alone. That is how connected our minds are to our sexuality. Research shows that women who fantasize have more satisfying orgasms and that fantasies help women become more aroused. You can use fantasy to add a little exciting boost, but stay present with the sensation in your body. If you stay in a fantasy in your head too long, there can be some disconnect between your body, your partner and your experience. A fantasy can help you orgasm for sure, but if you can connect the fantasy with your

Your Secret Chamber

partner, the pleasure will be higher. Smell him, touch him, and feel the details of your sensations. It is a better experience if your partner is fantasizing with you. Then you are more present with each other as you fantasize. If your partner ties you up he can say things like, "Now I get to have my way with you. You are under my control. I will make you scream for mercy." Or something like, "You were very naughty today girl. You should not try to escape me like that. See what I had to do to you because you disobeyed me? Now you will get it." Or whatever fantasy you are into. You could be his patient while he examines you, or vice versa. But if you participate together, then you can stay present, which is very important for great orgasms.

- **Open your throat**. Your throat is connected to your vagina. As you make noise, relax and open it. This actually opens your vagina more. Try this: put your fingers in your vagina and laugh, cough and say something loud. All of the above will cause the vaginal walls to squeeze. Open your throat by pressing your tongue against the floor of your mouth as hard as you can and your cervix will pull back and your vagina will open up. This is why it is important to not tense your jaw during orgasm or arousal. You can't open with your jaw locked. Let out big noises during orgasm and you will squeeze your partner even more while still allowing him to penetrate you deeply. If you keep your jaw and larynx tight you are limiting how deep your partner can penetrate you. Consciously relax your trachea. If your throat is sore after a great orgasm, then you may have held it too tight. Practice opening it and let out sounds with your neck and jaw relaxed.

Things that he can do to get you aroused:

- **Kissing.** Never underestimate kissing. Our mouths are linked directly with our sex organs. You can become very aroused by just kissing. If you are not getting turned on by kissing your partner, then tell him how you would like to be kissed. If he is kissing you, but not connected with you while he is doing it, then you may not enjoy the kissing. Men enjoy hearing what turns us on. If stated correctly, you can get exactly what you're asking for. Say something like, "You know what really turns me on? I love it when I feel connected to you when we kiss and you suck on the tip of my tongue." Or something like, "You know what really turns me on? I love it when you put your tongue in my mouth and I can suck on your soft tongue." Tell him what you like. If you don't know what you like, then spend some time thinking about it. Then have a passionate make out session. Spend twenty minutes just kissing. Soon you will be ripping each other's clothes off, although he will be ready after one long kiss.

- **He can caress you**. Ask him to touch your favorite place to be touched. Certainly you have places that work better than others to get you aroused. Do you know where those places are? For example, maybe you like him to begin on your back with a soothing touch to relax you. Then he can slowly move down to your buttocks and thighs with a light, tickly touch. After a few minutes he can go to the inner thigh and inner buttocks and pretty quickly you are ready for action. Do you have a spot such as this? If you don't know, then find out. Experiment with touch. Don't have him go straight for your hot buttons, like nipples and clit unless you are ready for that. If you are not in the mood, start with him caressing your

Your Secret Chamber

back in a sensual but non-sexual way. Then turn over when you're ready for the front.

- **He can give you a sensual and erotic massage.** Massage can begin non-sexual and then continue to the next level where it turns into caressing in more sensitive areas. This could go on and on until soon you are attacking each other. Tell him what feels good if he is not on the right track.
- **Have him kiss your neck, shoulders, tummy and other soft parts.**
- **Allow him to give you oral sex.** If you have a hang-up about receiving oral sex, you will serve yourself best by letting this one go. It could become one of your greatest pleasures. The clitoris has eight thousand nerve endings. That is a lot of pleasure in one little spot. Some of the keys to enjoying this are to open your hips wide and move your hips as you feel pleasure. Ask him to use his fingers to penetrate you. He can even stimulate your anus while his hand is right there, so close. Don't worry about if you ejaculate on him. He wants to cum on your face and in your mouth, so he won't mind if you do the same to him. Perhaps you are self-conscious and worry

Your Secret Chamber

about your smell. Most likely your man loves your smell and it isn't bad at all. You might even learn to enjoy the taste. After he kissed your lower lips, have him kiss your mouth. That taste is the taste of sex. It is delicious and erotic. If you do have a bad smell, it is due to diet, hygiene and health, so see a doctor or improve your diet.

- **Gaze into your eyes**. Connect with your partner. It will help you get aroused.
- **Have him lie on top of you and press his body against your open pelvis** without penetrating you. If you're not quite ready for sex, just lie in this position and hold each other. It will bring on wonderful sensations.
- **He can give you clitoral stimulation**. It may take you a long time to orgasm from just vaginal penetration. You may think that you can't do it. I find that difficult to swallow. You are built to orgasm from penetration. However, if you are not climaxing from penetration then additional stimulation is all that is usually necessary. That means stimulating the clitoris, nipple, anus, buttocks, biting your ear, or kissing. You may prefer a lot of

clitoral stimulation during penetration. Unless, of course, you just had a clitoral orgasm and want to rest the clit. Cock rings work very well for clit stimulation during intercourse. They are easy to find at your local sex toy shop. Men generally enjoy them also. But keep in mind that if your man is young and hasn't learned how to sustain his erection for a long time, so you have time to come, then the cock ring might make him cum even faster. Bummer. In that case he can use his hand, although that can get uncomfortable for you.

- **He can do breast stimulation**. Having your nipples in a man's mouth while he penetrates you is very tantalizing and often is just the push necessary to get you over that edge. This works well when you are on top and can dangle your beautiful breasts over his mouth. It also works when he is on top, as long as his neck works well and he can contort himself a little.
- **He can do anal stimulation**. Remember, the more areas that are electrified, the more turned on you will get. If you haven't tried this one, you are missing out. Researchers found that there are legs from the

Your Secret Chamber

clitoris that extend to the anus. If you want to maximize your orgasms, stimulation to this area will help. He can just reach around and touch the anus or he can insert a finger or two. This touch requires you to be quite aroused first. Touching around the anus for a while helps considerably, such as squeezing the buttocks. Whatever you are comfortable with is fine. Just remember to keep stretching that comfort level to reach higher and higher levels of pleasure. You may be comfortable trying anal sex or you may only be comfortable with a little finger stimulation. Just keep reaching for the most pleasure that you can enjoy. Remember to use lots of lubrication even with finger stimulation. Some couples feel comfortable with tongue action to the exterior of the anus or surrounding area. When it is clean, from a bath or thorough washing, this is safe. It is very erotic if you are comfortable trying this.

- **He can spank your buttocks.** I don't know why spanking feels so stimulating. Maybe it is because there is a correlation in the brain between pleasure and pain. Spanking feels exciting, erotic, and arousing and it bring lots of circulation and tingling to the pelvic floor. This doesn't work at all times. It works best if you are already excited, your lover is being passionate and you trust him. It also works well with a lot of massage to the buttock first. A loving partner will be careful not to hurt you. The idea is to stimulate the skin with a slight sting from the hand or whip. There are whips designed for this at the adult toy store that create many wonderful sensations. A long handled wooden spoon works excellent also. It is easy to manipulate without making it painful. After a little spanking, your pelvic floor will be tingling and ready for action.

- **Kissing while he penetrates you** helps you climax. The mouth and throat is tied to the vagina. Oral kissing stimulates many nerve endings and heightens your awareness of what is happening in your vagina.

- **He can use toys to arouse you.** There are toy store for kids and toys stores for grownups only. Don't be intimidated by them. They are your friend! When your man is far more stimulated than you are, and you want to catch up, have him use the vibrator on you. If you haven't done this before with your partner, you may be uncomfortable. You may be embarrassed to try it at first and don't see the value

Your Secret Chamber

of it. But the right toys can move you forward very quickly and add to your overall climax by making you more stimulated. It will also bond you together by opening both of you up to less inhibition with more communication. You will be surprised by how fun and easy it is to use toys together. If you live without children at home, the two of you could start the whole evening with the vibrator in the living room. He could just pull your pants down and start to stimulate you on the couch. Or lift your skirt and place the vibrator outside of your tights or panties. It could be like a fun game to start the mood flowing. You could even be cleaning up from dinner and he could bring the vibrator in to turn you on while you are at the sink. Pretty soon you are bent over the counter and he is pulling down your pants. You will want to go into the bedroom or else do it right in the kitchen. Toys offer variety to your love making. Men enjoy stimulation through variety. It is an important part of their make-up and explains why some men cheat. Your man doesn't experience multiple orgasms or the variety of orgasmic pleasures that you do. Every sexual experience can be different for us in sensations and satisfaction. For

Your Secret Chamber

men it all feels quite similar, only varying in intensity. So variety is the spice in sex for them. Get some ropes, a blindfold, a cock ring, a butt plug, or a glass dildo. A vibrator is a must have for you and all couples. Without it, you are simply missing out on great pleasure and bigger orgasms that you wouldn't miss if you knew about it. You won't use a vibrator all the time, but when you want it, it should be handy.

- **He can use a camera, video and mirrors to excite you.** It can be fun, playful and erotic to have your partner take digital photos of you in sexy, provocative positions. You can get turned on by being naked in front of the camera. You would be surprised how flattering the right angles and lighting can be. With digital you can always delete the ones you don't like or delete them all. Video is the same. He will love it and you can practice being very sexy. Don't be shy. You are sexy and beautiful. Show him what you've got! There is always the delete button if you worry about someone finding it. There are ways to keeping it safe for later viewing, if you are creative.

Your Secret Chamber

You may have a favorite position or role that you play with your lover. Perhaps you prefer being tied up, or you prefer being on top, or you like a certain role playing that you two do together. Maybe you like it when he touches you a certain way while you two are unwinding after dinner or you like him to rub your feet or tickle your shoulders. Let him know all of your preferences. These are very helpful when you are not particularly aroused. Your body will remember the way that it felt last time and it will trigger a natural response of excitement. You may like things that you can count on, like a certain touch that always makes you feel safe and sexy. Your man is usually seeking variety while you are looking for what is familiar. Let him know all of the familiar things that get you ready for lovemaking.

Your Secret Chamber

Sexercise: Do you know your body? Review the diagram below.

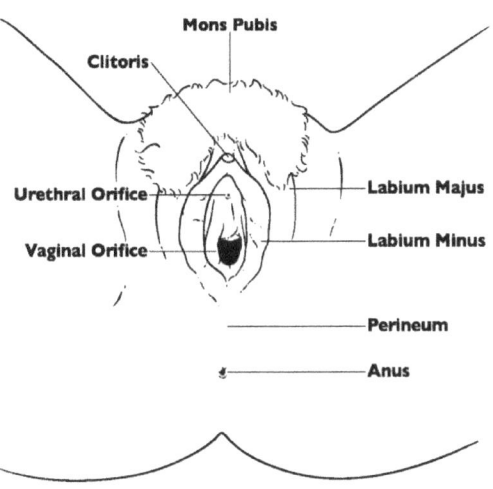

Sexercise:

List two new things you will do for yourself to get aroused prior to sex.

1.

2.

List two new things to get more aroused than you normally get prior to climax.

1.

2.

List two new things you will ask him to do for you.

1.

2.

Write about each experience and what you enjoyed or how you might change it for next time. Be specific so you learn from your new experience.

If you are struggling with getting aroused, consider the anatomy of your body. Not all women have the same sensitivity. If arousal or orgasm is difficult for you, consider ways to increase clitoral stimulation that are beyond what is listed here. Consider ice, a vibrator while using pressure, a strap on vibrator during intercourse, applying heat for a period of time to stimulate blood flow, or even piercing. Look into what works specifically for you.

Your Secret Chamber

Sexercise: Do the exercises above with your specific desires in mind. Write about your personal experience here that may be unique to you:

Set the stage. Have the best mood for cosmic orgasms in your bedroom.

Your bedroom is the place for inspiring pleasure, relaxation, trust and great sex. Look around and see how you can make it more sensual.

1. Keep the bedroom space clean, inspiring, and comfortable. Your bedroom is a retreat from the world where the two of you can relax and be totally intimate. If your room is filled with a project, paperwork or dirty laundry lying around, you will feel distracted from the moment. Hide away the distraction. Focus on the fun.
2. Keep the necessaries handy in the bedside table. It kills the mood to get up at the right moment and begin looking for the lubricant. Keep a sex mat handy so you won't worry about the mess on the sheets. Buy some nice massage oil. Keep

Your Secret Chamber

      something to wipe up with handy so you can lie together afterwards and cuddle in comfort.
3. Set the mood with romantic or exciting music.
4. Invest in a lamp that projects soft lighting. You will feel more beautiful with the right lighting.
5. Buy candles. Scented candles stimulate the senses, sooth and create a nice ambience.
6. Spoil yourself in your bedroom. Have a comfortable mattress with inviting sheets and coverings that you enjoy.
7. Buy some toys or erotica that you enjoy to spice things up.

Sexercise:

Invest in your orgasms.

Write down three improvements that you commit to making in your bedroom to help you want to spend more time there making love.

1.

2.

3.

Your Secret Chamber

We have talked about what you can do to take charge of your sexuality and be ready for mind blowing sex. Here is what your man can do for you to make it all come together.

What you want from your man for mind blowing orgasms:

1. For your man to care for you or to love you. This will be expressed by your man being helpful, lightening your load, or taking care of you in some way.
2. No pressure with ample time to allow you to get aroused
3. Being fully present and engaged with you, especially through eye contact.
4. Paying attention to what feels good to you and responding accordingly.
5. Whatever foreplay helps you get worked up prior to penetration: oral sex, lots of caressing, looking in your eyes, kissing, using a toy, clit stimulation and allowing you to climax one or more times before penetration. Refer to the list above for more ideas.

6. Long, sustained penetration, often with kissing, or breast, clit or buttock stimulation to bring you to a satisfying orgasm.
7. Patience. Women take much longer than a man.

If your total time in bed is taking less than thirty minutes and you are not having amazing orgasms, then have your man pay a lot of attention to this list. A mind-blowing orgasm can require one or two hours of wonderful lovemaking.

A note on erotica: There are many forms of erotica including steamy novels, movies, photographs, magazines, lingerie and sex toys. It is a multi-billion dollar annual industry. There are facts of nature that you can do nothing about, so you may want to stop resisting. *THE TELEGRAPH GROUP, The West Australian News* reported on December 3, 2009, 8:34 am that scientists at the University of Montreal launched a search for men who had never looked at pornography - but couldn't find any. Erotic pictures seem to be sought out universally by men. Other studies show that excessive use of pornography can have detrimental effects on committed relationships. Balance is helpful in all things. But if it is true that <u>all</u> men have viewed porn, then perhaps you shouldn't be angry if your partner decides to see some now and then.

Chapter 8
Mastering the Art of Orgasm

What constitutes an orgasm? Are they all the same?

Men and women experience all aspect of sex differently, including orgasm. Men's orgasms vary in intensity. You are fortunate because your orgasms can fluctuate in many respects.

- Female orgasms are multi-faceted experiences that differ greatly in pleasure and satisfaction. They change from day to day and vary from woman to woman.
- Women can enjoy one, two, ten or more orgasms in one love making experience.
- Women can enjoy orgasms that last for a few minutes, ten minutes or even more.
- Women can take orgasms to higher and higher stages of pleasure.

Your Secret Chamber

- Women can enjoy orgasms very late in life.
- After high arousal or several orgasms your cervix can lift out of the way and expose your fornix to your lover for mind blowing pleasure.

What does an orgasm feel like? How do I know that I've had one?

This may be a question from a young woman that is just beginning her sexual journey. Yet this question can also come from a woman who is having difficulty with orgasm and their sexual experiences. So let's talk about what an orgasm feels like.

There are many aspects to how an orgasm feels. They are not all the same. One constant with all orgasms is that the vaginal wall and pelvic floor contract and the feeling is very pleasurable. The contractions and enjoyment can happen even without an orgasm, when you become aroused. You can have strong contractions and not reach a peak. Reaching a peak of pleasure is the key to experiencing an orgasm.

When you reach an orgasm, you feel a build up towards it first, with pleasure getting stronger and stronger and your muscles getting tighter and tighter. You get lost in a whirlwind of sensations and pleasure swirling through your body. It can be described as a warm or tingly feeling in part or all of your body. You feel happy and your heart feels expanded. Often you feel love and intense desire for your partner. You want more and more of the bliss and joy. You feel like you can't get enough until finally the delight reaches a pinnacle where you enjoy a relief from the craving for more. At that point you reach the top of the orgasm build-up and you roll off the peak and the pleasure subsides. Desire is replaced with satisfaction.

 I will talk later about how that peak can last for a long time, ten minutes or longer, depending on how long you can physically keep contracting.

 Women describe the crest like going over the edge of a waterfall, or going out to the moon and back. A few women say it feels like they are going pee. Ejaculating from a G-spot orgasm feels closest to that description. Prior to orgasm pleasure builds to a point until it finally releases. Then you return to your previous state of less pleasure sensations with one exception, you are now more relaxed and have released a lot of tension and good hormones; the greater the build-up, the bigger the orgasm and release of tension.

Your Secret Chamber

After an orgasm you sometimes feel so overstimulated that you want a break from stimulating touch. Other times you want to keep going and ride the wave into the next orgasm. Sometimes you feel like you cannot move a single muscle. Generally if you can't move or you want a break, then it was a satisfying orgasm. Smaller ones, build to bigger ones, and leave you craving more. When you are satisfied sexually, you generally will know that you are done.

Sexual frustration

Before we go on, I want to address sexual frustration. If you are frustrated because you are not reaching orgasm, and you worry that you can't do it, let me reassure you. There are very few women who are completely unable to have an orgasm. Spending some time alone masturbating might relieve your fears quickly. Following the steps in this workbook will guide you to achieving sexual bliss. There is often an underlying problem that is causing the lack of orgasm, such as depression, health issues, fear of letting go, or lack of trust.

As I mentioned in earlier chapters, some women have fewer nerve ending throughout their pelvic region

Your Secret Chamber

or they may have a small clitoris that is buried and difficult to stimulate. In each of these cases a woman may go to further extremes to become stimulated enough to orgasm.

In most cases you have enough nerves endings accessible but there must be adequate time for stimulation, which is nearly always far more than your man thinks is necessary. **Consistency is important while building to orgasm. Have your lover focus the same amount of pressure and angle for several minutes while you build to a peak. Communicate to your lover when you want him to stay constant.** Sometime he changes angles to prevent himself from climaxing. Detailed communication is the best way to work through these differences.

If your man is one who comes quickly and then he is done and not willing to bring you to orgasm, then sit down with him and have some serious communication. That is unacceptable in the world of feminine pleasure. Most men desire to be a good lover. Most men know that pleasing you gives them great satisfaction. <u>What they may not know is that the better time that you have, the more that you will want sex.</u> Talk to your partner. Tell him that if he finishes quickly, then he must turn his attention to pleasing you. And although you will prefer a hard cock inside you, if he has come, then there are other ways that he can please you. He can use his fingers, mouth or a toy. The point is if you are left sexually frustrated, you will not be dragging him back in the bedroom for more of that tomorrow night.

Other causes of lack of orgasm could be hang-ups, not knowing your body, health problems, and tension or being stuck in your head. Review the previous chapters regarding these issues. It's almost certain that you are capable of having orgasms.

Types of Orgasms

Let's get down to the nitty gritty. Please put on your bedroom ear and eyes...we are going to talk about the fundamentals, including details about sex. The information is not for weak eyes. If you want to get good at sex, get comfortable talking about it.

> "I was amazed at how much more powerful I felt when I learned that I should use sexy language with my boyfriend. I told him that I was thinking about his cock and he loved it. After we made love I told him what I liked and what I wanted to try next time. Now I feel so much more relaxed about sex and it's more fun." G

Seeking a Variety of Orgasms

You have many erogenous zones. They are worth exploring. We will concentrate on the major zones that will allow you to build your orgasms to the next level.

My goal in this workbook, and the courses that I teach, is to help you become comfortable experiencing pleasures and realize the benefits of deep penetration with richly satisfying orgasms. I will discuss how to achieve the other types, but most orgasms are a prelude to the ultimate goal. You can use all of the other orgasms to walk you up the ladder to the big bang! If

Your Secret Chamber

you can practice these activities with a willing partner, you can achieve unfathomable bliss.

The list of potential pleasures is extremely extensive so I will only list some of the main ways you can become aroused and the potential orgasms you can enjoy, starting with some of the lower levels of pleasure and working up to the higher ones.

Over the Waterfall: Making Out:

Kissing is a great way to get the sexual juices flowing. Your mouth is often your first introduction to sexual pleasure. Enjoying an orgasm with kissing and touching is easier with a brand new partner whom you are very attracted to and super aroused with or if you are young and haven't had naked time with your partner. With a partner you know well, you will be tempted to move the love making forward, so making out may not last long enough to have an orgasm. Yet it is definitely possible if you take the time.

To maximize oral stimulation, have your partner take the tip of your tongue in his mouth while he sucks on the tip and circles it in both directions with his tongue. Have him do this for two full minutes or more.

Your Secret Chamber

This indirectly stimulates your clitoris and, if he is present and connected with you, it can give you an orgasm. You will have to stick your tongue out enough that he can take it into his mouth.

Now have him present his tongue into your mouth. Suck on as much of his tongue as you can reach. Do not suck so hard that you pull his tongue away from the back of his mouth. That will hurt him. Suck it without pulling. Notice how his tongue feels in your mouth. It feels similar to his cock. Do this action for a minute or two and he will certainly get hard and you will feel the indirect stimulation in your vagina. Then let him do the same action to your tongue with his mouth.

Random tongue action does not produce the same arousal that these focused tongue actions do. He won't have an orgasm from them, but you might. You will want to do these same tongue actions during penetration to enhance both of your orgasms.

Intense kissing, while he lies on top of you thrusting you without penetration can cause an orgasm. If he presses his hard cock against your pelvis, both of you can have a release just from the pressure and friction. Most likely this will just get you aroused. The more you connect well during the kissing, the more aroused you will get.

Through the Roof: Breast stimulation with mouth:

It is amazing how wonderful it feels to have the breast stimulated. I've heard many women state that they don't enjoy nipple stimulation or that it does nothing for them. If you are one of those women, don't give up on your nipples. You can train them for ultimate pleasure.

The nipples are a curious part of our bodies. They don't enjoy being stimulated in all circumstances and most of the time you will have to be turned on to appreciate the sensations that comes from the nipples. There are various ways that you can learn to enjoy your nipples. The nipples do not generally like to be grabbed directly, unless you are already quite turned on. If you are still working your way up to turned on, then:

- The nipple should be approached gradually. He should start by kissing your neck. If your neck is ticklish, then you are not excited yet, or you do not trust your partner.

Your Secret Chamber

- Another subtle approach to the nipple is to gently handle the entire breast, avoiding pinching or rubbing the nipple directly. That indirect pressure will help get the nipple ready for action.
- If you are still unable to participate with pleasure from your nipples, then play with them yourself when you are already aroused. Do what feels good and get them ready for his lips.
- Once they are ready and excited, and then allow your partner to **lick your nipples**. Gradually your partner can **suck, bite gently and pull on them**. A **rapid licking or generous sucking** over a period of time will create a nipple orgasm. It is worth getting them in the game.

Here are some hints to help it happen.

- It helps if there is pressure against your pelvis. Your clothes can be on or off. But his body should be pressed against your labia with good pressure.

  You can do this same scenario with penetration, but that is not a nipple orgasm which we are talking about now. A nipple orgasm is a great way to get off without penetration if you are avoiding it for some reason. Mostly this kind of orgasm is a prelude to more because it is not very satisfying. It just feels good.

Another helpful hint is:

- Try having your arms restrained while he kisses your breasts. He can hold your hands above your head so that you cannot move them or he can tie them so his hands are free. This will heighten your pleasure because it increases your ability to submit to him. Surrendering also allows you to let go and enjoy more. I will speak of surrendering often because it is one of the most important aspects of the ultimate orgasm. If you can have your hands tied in this situation, you are on your way to allowing your partner to take you while you give up control.

Note:

This is not a lesson in being tickled. If your partner ever takes the opportunity to tie you up and tickle you, communicate firmly that you will not agree to bondage unless it feels good. Never allow your partner to do any activity that does not feel good to you, or you cannot easily tolerate, just so that he can cum. Otherwise you won't trust enough to let go and you won't be excited to come back.

- While you are contracting during this orgasm, your vagina has nothing to squeeze against. This is part of the reason this orgasm is not satisfying and will leave you wanting more, which is perfect for building you up to the next level.

Tickle My Backside: Stimulation to thighs, buttocks and outside area of labia

This is a toss-up with nipple stimulation. Nipple stimulation is much more intense, but I listed this one next because it can be a more satisfying type of orgasm. This works very well if you are not in the mood and want help getting there.

You might want to be tied up in this situation, because again, it forces vulnerability, which takes you to deeper and deeper levels of surrender. Bondage, however, is not necessary to enjoy this and you can learn to surrender fully without ever being tied up.

Fully undressed, lie face down or face up; preferably do one and then the other. Close your eyes

Your Secret Chamber

and allow your partner to caress you. You may ask him to begin with your back and slowly work his way to your buttocks and thighs. Communicate with him the pressure that feels good to you.

Allow your partner to move his touch to the inner area of your thighs. For this orgasm he can touch you everywhere except extended touch to the clitoris or any vaginal penetration. This is another rung on the ladder of pleasure. If he wants to rub your clit for a quick O, remind him of the goal, which is to build arousal. He should enjoy this as well, because he gets to look at and touch your body while he can watch your response and build your excitement. In order for you to reach a climax, this will either take a long while or he can increase the pressure on your labia and inner thighs. He must use lubrication if he does lots of stimulation to the labia. He can take the labia lips in his finger and massage them. This will feel amazing. He can use a finger or two to caress the inside of the labia without penetrating the vagina. Have him hold your buttocks with the other hand or stroke your inner thigh. Also ask him to put firm pressure with his fingers all around your labia on the pelvic floor bones. Direct pressure to this area is highly stimulating.

Once you are sufficiently aroused, then you can turn over so he can lie on you and move his hips without penetrating you. You will be able to have a small orgasm from that if he has aroused you. He will get aroused and want to penetrate you. His goal is always to penetrate. Remind him that building up your arousal is the goal so that the energy is huge and ultimately the release is too. Your arousal will also increase the bonding between you two. It will cause you to squeeze your vaginal muscles and be more active, which will increase his pleasure as well.

Spank Me Baby: External stimulation to the anus

The anus is a well-kept secret. Perhaps you have taboos regarding sex, especially anal sex, thinking that it is dirty, or sinful. In regards to anal sex you might feel that good girls don't do that. If you don't have any interest in anal stimulation, consider how you think about it. Do you feel it is dirty? Are you embarrassed? There isn't any area of your body that should not be touched by a caring partner, especially if it feels good.

Your Secret Chamber

It is not necessary to participate in anal stimulation to reach the ultimate orgasm. However, experiencing as much pleasure as possible, knowing your body well and what feels good, as well as building up your arousal in every way that you can, all contribute to the success of your best orgasm.

Here is a gentle guide to opening this doorway of pleasure. If you are new to this idea, begin by allowing your partner to caress your buttocks. Have him take his time. If you are self-conscious about your derriere then work on the chapter about loving your body. He should do this touch in a dimly lit room to help enhance the shadow and outline of your sexy bottom.

Take five, ten or more minutes to let this pleasure build. As he rubs your cheeks, allow him to spread your legs and rub in the crease of your butt cheeks. The more caresses to the buttocks, the more ready your anus is for touch. Spanking works well here too for extra stimulation. He will want to go faster than you, so encourage him to slow down. As he approaches the anus, focus on the sensation. It is a very nice sensation, especially the more aroused that you are. When he goes for direct contact with the anus, be sure he is using lubricant on his finger, even on the outside.

Your Secret Chamber

The anus does not make its own lube, and it doesn't feel good dry.

Allow him to simply touch it and rub it back and forth with his finger. If it feels really good, and you are aroused from it, you could allow him to insert his finger about one inch, or much more if you want. He can also rub your anus like a clitoris and bring you to orgasm. It will be a short, quick unsatisfying orgasm that will leave you very turned on and wanting much more. Once you learn to enjoy this touch, you can experiment with more penetration.

REMEMBER:
- Use ample lubrication
- Penetrate super slowly. Take two to three full minutes to fully penetrate with a penis.
- The more stimulated that you are the better
- The more touching of the buttocks and close proximity to the anus the better. It helps to do this stimulation for ten minutes or longer.
- Spanking can be very helpful

Your Secret Chamber

Deep Throat: Giving oral sex to a man

Are you aware of the extreme pleasure that you can receive from giving your man fellatio. The penis feels amazing on your lips, tongue, inside your mouth and throat. It is soft and offers many sensations.

Here are some helpful hints:

- Decide the position that works best for you. It is nice to have the option to look into your partner's eyes while doing it so you can connect with him and watch his face as you pleasure him. He will think that it is very sexy as he watches his cock move in and out of your mouth. Another great position is 69, with his mouth on your clit and labia. You can also turn your body so that his hand can reach your bottom and clit so he can touch you while you use your mouth on him.
- Once you know your position, then tell your partner that you are going to just enjoy his cock. This is not about him, but about you. You are not going to make him cum, but you might cum. You want him hard for more play later. You are

just getting both of you excited. Tell him to hold his cum.

- Now, roll his cock against your face. Feel how smooth and soft it is. Feel it with your checks. Now smell it. Inhale that beautiful scent of maleness, your partners scent. Let that smell permeate you. Enjoy it. Tell him, "I love your dick."

- Now slowly, gently, kiss his cock, then allow your tongue to taste it and feel it. Lick the underside of his shaft at the base of the head. That is a sensitive spot.

- Hold his cock firm with one hand, as you lick around it. Let it get wet with your saliva. Wet feels the best to him and it will help you enjoy it as well. Never mind the mess. Sex is messy.

- When you are ready, open your mouth and receive the head of his penis. Lick it while it is in your mouth. Move your tongue around. He will like that. Close your eyes for a moment and be present with this delicious part of your partner. Enjoy it. Revel in it. Breathe in. Sigh. Connect with your partner. Pay attention to what he likes and how he reacts. Look at him when you can. Let him know that you are enjoying this.

- Push the head of the penis against the inside of your cheek. Let the pressure of your cheek stimulate his head. Do that on the other side. Alternate back and forth, one side then the other. Suck as you slowly withdraw his penis. Consume it again and suck as you pull it out.

- Allow his head to rub against the roof of your mouth. Notice how that feels. Enjoy it. The roof of your mouth is like the G-spot in the vagina. With consistent rubbing and pressure you can become very aroused and even cum. Do this for a little while. Enjoy the pleasure.

- <u>Slowly</u>, <u>slowly</u>, allow his cock to go further and further into your throat. Some days this will be easier than other days. It helps if you start this when he is not as hard and it slowly gets harder so you can have time to have him deep in your throat when the head is not as big. Practice pressing your tongue hard against the floor of your mouth to open your throat. You may not be able to do this, but I hope that you will be able to

Your Secret Chamber

open yourself this much and allow yourself to be deeply penetrated.

- <u>Do the same motion consistently, allowing the penis to rub on areas of your mouth and throat that feel good. With repeated action, you can orgasm.</u>

Secret: There is a point, deep in your throat, beyond your gag reflex that feels like you are actually being penetrated in the vagina as it is stroked. Amazing orgasms happen when you are able to reach this point. You may not reach the full orgasm, but you will be much more aroused from doing deep throat action. It will get you ready for full penetration. The orgasms from this are short, but quite satisfying because you are being penetrated.

Sexercise: Practice this pleasure with your partner. Have you had a great experience with deep throat penetration? Yes   No (circle one) If yes, how did it go?

Did you feel yourself becoming aroused as you enjoyed his dick in your mouth? Yes No (circle one)

Your Secret Chamber

Faster, Faster: Fingers to clitoris

To yourself: Did you know that the clitoris has eight thousand nerve endings? No wonder it feels so good. Yet finger stimulation to the clit generally has a short peak and does not provide the full-body satisfaction and bonding of penetration. It may, however, be the most common orgasm that you have. If you are not communicating with your lover, you are not likely reaching great orgasms during intercourse. The result can be that you must create your own climax. That wouldn't be such a sad problem, if it weren't for the fact that self-stimulation to the clitoris is usually a quick peak with a fast drop off and not nearly as satisfying as an orgasm from penetration with your partner. Not to mention that a bonding orgasm with a lover gives us so much more satisfaction than self-stimulation can. The best orgasms that you can obtain rush through your whole body providing pleasure on a larger scale. But let's not knock it. The clitoral orgasm is the fastest, easiest orgasm to obtain. If you are having any difficulty having an orgasm, start here. There is definitely a level of satisfaction from this orgasm.

Your Secret Chamber

The keys to giving yourself a clitoral jump are lubrication and fast movement. Vibrators work quickly and avoid cramping up your hand. Preferably get a vibrator that can penetrate you while stimulating your clit at the same time. That will put you on a fast track to pleasurable contractions and then relaxation. One of the more versatile vibrators is the Jack Rabbit. It is also water proof and can be used in the bath tub. A section of the shaft is packed with small metal balls that spin under the front half of the rubbery cock, granting more stimulation while two small rabbit ears vibrate on the clit. You will have an orgasm in no time at all.

The clitoris can become hypersensitive after a clit orgasm, yet it should get you ready so that pressure from his pelvic bone against you during penetration will continue to stimulate the clit just right. If you want a break, you can either wait to rest the clit, or do other activities that leave the clit alone for a while. One last note; you may feel a point where you don't think that you can take anymore stimulation to the clit, like you are done enjoying the pleasure. Push beyond that feeling whenever you can. Lighten up on the pressure is necessary, but continue to roll with the intense pleasure.

There is more pleasure waiting for you on the other side of that feeling.

From a man: Your man can use his hands or any of the toys available for this purpose. Let him know that consistent pressure and motion make it happen for you. If you really enjoy clitoral stimulation, I recommend trying a vibrating cock ring. The ring fits around your partner's penis and it vibrates on your clit while your lover penetrates you. Keep good communication while he touches your clit. Tell him what feels good to you.

Wrap My Legs Around You: Receiving oral sex

Receiving oral sex may be your favorite stimulation if you are comfortable with your body. Oral sex offers a lot of stimulation which makes reaching orgasm easy. Oral sex is an excellent prelude to intercourse as it heightens your arousal and prepares you for a bigger, more satisfying orgasm. With all of that clitoral and labial stimulation, you will welcome penetration and his body pressure will continue to stimulate the clitoris.

Your Secret Chamber

If you are uncomfortable with the idea of your lover's mouth on your privates, then I suggest taking a few steps to help you through this phobia. Oral sex should be very satisfying for you and your man. It is sensual, tender and bonding for both of you. It is one of the most intimate, revealing, personal and vulnerable things that you can do together. There are fewer ways that you can get closer to your partner.

If you are healthy, then your vaginal juices are quite tasty to your lover. Feel free to taste your own juices. This idea may seem strange at first, but it is good for you to be comfortable with your taste, so that your lover may kiss your mouth after he has kissed you elsewhere or so you can be comfortable preforming oral sex on him after he has penetrated you. One very sexy idea is to have your lover insert his fingers into your vagina and then allow you to lick his fingers. It will be sexy to him and it may even get you more aroused.

You may also use oral sex as just foreplay. It is not necessary to climax to build you closer to the big one. If your lover licks you slowly, and doesn't focus on the clitoris, then you are likely to just build your excitement, rather than release it. Practicing not releasing when an orgasm seem imminent is an excellent way to build the energy up in order to heighten things, since the biggest orgasms come from a great deal of sexual tension.

As the energy and excitement build-up, pull the excitement up into your body towards your heart and head. You are spreading the intensity from being concentrated on one area to being incorporated into the whole body. This will create a euphoria of pleasure throughout your body. Spreading the excitement does several things for you:

- It allows you to prolong the pleasure before orgasm.
- It allows you to experience the pleasure more full-body.
- It increases the amount of explosion you will be able to experience.
- It allows you to get in touch with the powerful energy center of your body.

In my follow-up course I talk about how to use this energy to direct creative energy towards things that you want to accomplish in life, and how to merge your feelings with your partner's.

Your Secret Chamber

Sexercise: Receive oral sex while you are on your hands and knees or you are bent over the counter and he is behind you.

Do you Feel Me? Finger and toy penetration with ample lubrication

Fingers have one advantage that the penis doesn't have. Fingers can more easily feel a certain location to focus a lot of stimulation, like the g-spot. You have many wonderful stimulation points within the vagina, all of which produce different sensations and different types of orgasms. With the cooperation of your partner, you can explore the many different places that feel good and notice the changing sensations and the orgasms that result. Once he can find those places with his fingers, he can eventually find them with his penis.

Sexercise: When you are very aroused, and have done a few of the other stimulating foreplay activities:

1. Ask your partner to insert his fingers inside you and focus the tip of his fingers on certain spots. Have him find the G-spot and stroke it with pressure. Once he is familiar with how it feels and where it is

Your Secret Chamber

located, he can find it easier with the head of his penis and focus some pressure on it when he is inside you.

2. Have your partner insert two fingers inside you and notice what happens when you laugh, cough, sneeze or talk loud. He will feel your vaginal muscles contract. Also have him feel what happens when you do a Kegel exercise.

3. Have your partner stroke the cervix, stroking it with the top of his finger. This also feels very nice and can produce a unique orgasm.

4. Ask him to focus on the opening of the vagina, inserting several fingers about three inches in a rhythmic fashion. Consistent rhythm makes a big difference here. Use lubrication.

5. See how far your partner can penetrate you with his fingers. See if he can reach deep inside you. Experiment with lying in different positions that allow him more access. Open yourself up to him. Allow his hand to really enter you. Can he reach your fornix vault, the very back of your vagina?

6. Have him feel your vagina to find the cervix. Have him notice how far the cervix is protruding into your vagina. Have him check this again after you have

had some orgasms and have become highly aroused. He should notice that you have opened up, the cervix has pulled back and Your Secret Chamber is accessible.

NOTES:

If he puts his index and middle finger inside you with his palm up and bends his fingers slightly, he should be right on the g-spot. It feels like a firm, bumpy patch in the vagina.

The cervix is located further back. It feels like the end of your nose. He should not hit this hard, but stroke it gently.

Around the World: Anal penetration with ample lubrication

You may never become comfortable with anal penetration. Do not be surprised if that is how you feel right now. Once again I will say that this is not required to reach the big O. If you decide to participate, it is an exciting, occasional pleasure done when you are in the mood for more penetration. Even if you are comfortable with this idea, most likely you will not be interested in it very often.

Your Secret Chamber

With that being said, it is certainly worth exploring. You and your man have sexually arousing areas in and around the anus. It is the way that our bodies are designed. Who are we to argue with nature?
Sexercise: Pick up a <u>vibrating</u> toy made specifically for anal penetration at your local sex shop. If you are too embarrassed to buy it, let your partner do it. He will love the idea, most likely. In general men are not as reserved about sex as women.

Start by being very clean. The drug stores carry disposable enemas which help if you are feeling not empty.

Allow your partner to stimulate the outside of your anus with his lubricated finger or a lubricated toy. He should start with a buttock massage first. When you are aroused from his touch, let him know by arching your back and pressing your buttock upwards. Or you can tell him when you are ready. Allow him to stimulate the anus and then insert the toy slowly with lube. It will feel strange at first, especially for the first inch. Just allow that feeling. Once the toy is further inserted, it should feel nice. Allow him to move the device in and out. Again, this will feel strange at first, but after a few minutes it feels exciting and arousing. With a four inch or longer toy or a man's penis you can have a nice orgasm from this stimulation. Or it could just build things towards the big O.

Some men have very large dicks that are difficult to accept in the anus. If your partner has a very large cock, you could take it in. It is physically possible, but it can be difficult to enjoy. It can also cause tearing, pain and swelling. If he is very large, then I suggest that you stick with the toy; no pun intended. For large to average size, a toy that is small at the tip and gradually gets larger helps get you ready for his cock to penetrate you.

For anal penetration with a cock several things are important to note. First use lots and lots and lots of lubrications. Use a condom if you do not know the status of your partner. Blood born STD's are transferred easily this way. Your partner must go extremely slow. He will always want to go much faster than you are ready for. It should take a full two to three minutes to insert the penis. Also the penis must be very hard. A soft penis will not go in. Lastly, you should push against him, not retract. Think open and relax. This is a great exercise in allowing your partner to penetrate you while you relax and accept.

It is also nice to use a toy in the anus while your partner penetrates you vaginally. Being filled up this full heightens your pleasure.

Open Me Up: Vaginal penetration not too deep and not focused on the G-spot

The opening of your vagina is highly sensitive. With <u>consistent</u> stimulation, a wonderful orgasm can be produced that leaves you building up to craving deeper penetration. You can accomplish this orgasm by having your partner penetrate you very shallowly with quick movements back and forth. He will be very tempted to go in deeper, so be sure to communicate with him that this is temporary and deeper penetration will be forthcoming.

This orgasm will require consistent movement for several minutes. He should stimulate your clitoris slightly at the same time either by lying on you or lightly touching the clitoris with his fingers. Or he can stimulate your nipples with his tongue or fingers. This orgasm feels very nice but will leave you wanting more penetration.

G-Licious: Vaginal penetration with focus on the G-spot

We talked about where the G-spot is within the vagina. When stimulated for an extended period of time you can have one of the most satisfying of all of the orgasms. The G-spot orgasm often produces a full-body pleasure all by itself without it being necessary to pull the energy up through your body. Be sure to have your man focus on the same place that feels good until you orgasm. If he changes angles or pressure, you will lose your build up.

This type of orgasm usually feels like someone has plugged you into a light socket so that electricity is surging through your body. The G-spot also has glands within the area that produce female cum. When this area is stimulated for enough time to produce a G-spot orgasm, then you can ejaculate cum. The amount can be a teaspoonful or up to a full cup, creating quite a mess.

Female Ejaculation. You may be self-conscious about ejaculation, because of the mess; but it doesn't smell and it dries eventually. **A good way to address this concern is with a mat that is absorbent.** Purchase a plastic backed baby sheet and cut it into squares, sew the edges and place under you. Then you can let go without worry. The mat is very portable too.

Ejaculation is quite satisfying. If you haven't experienced it, it feels most similar to peeing. You know the feeling you get when you have held your pee for a long time and you finally get to go? It feels like that only one hundred times better. Instead of contracting, the vagina actually pushes outward. Fluid from the glands at the G-spot spills out in small or large quantities. Get your man to master giving you this and you will want one of these every night.

Ejaculation will occur when your vaginal muscles push out, rather than squeeze inward. It is the difference in how you use your vaginal muscles that allows the juices to flow out. You can consciously push out or pull in depending on whether or not you wish to enjoy this wet release.

Sexercise: Try many new positions to add variety to your love making and notice the new stimulation for both of you. Many positions do not put the right pressure on the clitoris, so purchase a strap on clit stimulator so that you are happy in all positions. List the new positions that you tried and which ones that worked well for you.

1.
2.
3.

Sexercise: Choose at least three lighter orgasms or pleasures to enjoy prior to any penetration. Build to full arousal where you crave penetration before you allow it. Write about your experience here.

Sexercise: Seduce your lover by making him want you. Text him suggestive things such as what you want to do to his body. Dress provocatively. Tease him. Make him want you until he can't wait any longer. This should make you highly aroused. Write about your experience here.

Sexercise: Try building up to one of the really big orgasms. Work your way up slowly by getting highly

Your Secret Chamber

aroused and doing several small orgasms first. As you build towards orgasm stay relaxed and let it overtake you. Try different things like squeezing the pelvic floor and then relaxing it. Try opening your throat to allow for deeper penetration. Spread the pleasure through your body. Write about your experience here.

Sexercise:

Write a note to your man and tell him what turns you on, but keep it short. You don't want him climbing into bed with a laundry list of do's and don'ts. If you have a lot to say, tell him more when he has mastered a few of your requests. Use the language that men enjoy. It may seem strange or unromantic to you, but that is part of embracing sexiness. This language is the language of sex. Learn to speak it with your lover. Example:

Hello my King!

I am looking forward to making love with you tonight. I want to tell you about a few things that really

Your Secret Chamber

turn me on and a few things that I want us to do together.

It makes me wet and horny when you look into my eyes while you are penetrating me hard, thrusting and thrusting me. I want you to put your tongue in my mouth so that I can suck on it and savor it. I want your dick sliding in and out of my mouth and way into my throat. I am going to orgasm from you penetrating my throat and filling me up as full as possible.

I look forward to you licking me and tasting my love juices. Then I want to taste those yummy juices when you kiss me. There is nothing that I don't want to try with you. There is no part of my body that you can't have. I am all yours baby. Take me!!!!

I am at home wanting you and waiting to be satisfied by your hard dick, strong arms and warm lips. Your horny girl,
Jen

This letter is exactly what a man wants to hear. He will listen to this language and it will register with him. So if you want to communicate what you want in bed, use words he enjoys or he might forget. When you speak to your girlfriends you can be less direct, but not

Your Secret Chamber

with a man. They don't connect the dots the way women do. Tell him directly with erotic words and you will get what you want. Always refer to his penis with sexy words. The word cock or dick works best with men.

Write your letter here for practice. Then write it in a nice card or on paper and give it to him, soon!

Chapter 9
Going Deep

If deep penetration is difficult for you, it may be because you have resistance and barriers to receiving your lover in the deepest possible way. Why is that? It's the same reason that you may have your hearts closed to deep, unconditional love, the same reason you are not authentic with friends and lovers, and why you don't tell our partner when something is bothering you; you are afraid. Fear may be stopping you every day from the best sex of your life.

Deep penetration means being your most vulnerable, physically and sexually. If you are in love with your partner, then it means being the most vulnerable emotionally also. It is the deepest physical connection you can make with your man. He enters your body, your cavity, and the deeper he is inside you, the more connected you are. Being totally open is the most you can offer your lover.

Your Secret Chamber

So how do you go deep? If you have been doing the sexercises up to this point, then you are working toward this goal. Going deep is about trust, blossoming, being open, being aroused, and vulnerability, as well as allowing and receiving.

- Trust your partner and yourself to keep you safe in every way.
- Blossom into the amazing woman that you are without holding any of yourself back.
- Be open to what happens, open to your partner, and open to sexuality and connecting.
- Be vulnerable emotionally, physically and sexually.
- Become sexually excited. Let it build and build.
- Allow your partner to take you, to direct you, to penetrate you, and to please you.
- Receive his advancement, his penetration, his gift of pleasure and his focus on you.

Your Secret Chamber

Why is deep penetration important? Can I have a heavenly orgasm without going deep?

There are advantages to deep penetration. Yes, you can have amazing orgasms without being penetrated past your cervix. But think of this; if your lover put his dick inside you only one inch, and that is as far as he would go, what would you tell him? "Go deeper." If he penetrated you exactly two inches what would you say? "Go deeper." Hopefully you are getting the picture. Deeper is better! The further he is inside your vagina, the more stimulation that you are getting at once.

Additionally, as you become more open sexually, you will become more open as a woman to your unique authentic inner radiance. If you allow your lover to access Your Secret Chamber, he will access deep parts of you that you didn't find on your own.

More good news is that there are wonderful nerve endings at the back of your vagina. Yeah! Additionally as his cock slides past your cervix, you are stimulated even more from all of the nerve endings on your cervix.

You may resist this idea of deep because you have had intercourse where your lover hit your cervix and you experienced pain. So now you believe that deep

Your Secret Chamber

is painful. Deep can be painful if you are not aroused enough. The cervix does not like to be hit with the head of the penis. It hurts, no doubt. A direct hit can shift your mood quickly. So going deep requires that you be very aroused, vulnerable and trusting so that your cervix will pull up out of the way. It may also require you to adjust positions. Even when you are aroused and the cervix is pulled back, the cervix can still be hit when you are in certain positions.

When you are having an orgasm the cervix will even bob up and down as you contract. Amazing. Going deep is similar to going deep with a blow job. You have to work up to it and be aroused so that you will open and receive him.

If you are experiencing just a slight discomfort from the cervix getting bumped a little, see if you can relax and accept that little pain as if it is a pleasure. Deciding not to resist can shift the pain into pleasure and move the cervix out of the way even more. The cervix is an erogenous zone that enjoys being touched.

Hints to finding the gold:
1. Begin slowly at a comfortable amount of penetration when you are excited from foreplay.

Your Secret Chamber

2. Gradually increase how deep your partner is penetrating you. Remember that what gradual means to you may different from what gradual means to your partner. Men tend to go faster than us. Communicate with him what you want.
3. Focus your body on relaxing, opening, trusting and seeking pleasure from letting go.
4. Try different hip angles or body positions with your partner to open up the area and allow the penis to slide past the cervix into the vault. There are excellent wedges that you can purchase to help with comfortable positions that enhance going deep.
5. Blossom, think open. Open your legs more. Feel deep into your vagina and clear the way with your intention.
6. Continue to communicate. You will probably enjoy having the penetration at the deepest point to be held for a second or two. You will have to request this because the man is thinking about stimulation from movement. For you, however, that deep place feels great, so you will want the feeling to linger at that wonderful spot for additional stimulation. The man will be happy to

Your Secret Chamber

linger a second or two when the end of your vagina squeezes the head of his penis, which happens when you get very stimulated from him pausing deep inside you. An added benefit of having him pause is that it should help hold off his pending ejaculation so that you can receive the extra stimulation you need to have a huge orgasm. He is less stimulated when he is not moving.

Note: In most cases his penis size will not matter. Your vagina can contract around a finger or two when fully aroused. It can certainly be filled up by a penis of most any size. Go as deep as you can with your partner.

Sexercises: Go for the deepest penetration that you have ever experienced. Do the following:

- Set aside some time for some love making. One to two hours is an excellent amount of time. You can take your time and let things develop. Begin early so that you don't get tired. If you have kids at home, do the best you can. Consider hiring a babysitter to take the kids out.

- Open yourself up to your partner by feeling yourself let go, become highly aroused and give way for him to really see you and enter you fully. Let go of thoughts about your body, the kids, your 'To Do List' or tomorrow's agenda. Be present in that moment. Connect with your partner; make eye contact, feel him. Breathe from your heart; open your heart. Open, open, open; let go of everything unrelated to that moment with your lover.

- Move in different positions if you are having difficulty getting past the cervix. The more aroused you are, and the more open and vulnerable you feel, the easier it will be. Try some of the many different arousal methods mentioned in an earlier chapter so that your cervix will lift out of the vagina and open up Your Secret Chamber.

- When your partner has penetrated you fully, and you feel that sensation at the back of your vagina, ask him to pause there briefly on each push forward. That small pause causes a bit more simulation on that area. It is just what helps to push you over the orgasm edge. Ask him to keep doing this until you cum. It may take several

Your Secret Chamber

minutes. If you are getting close, but not reaching climax, that could mean two things. You are either not relaxed enough, or you desire additional stimulation. Have your partner kiss you or stimulate your nipples or anus while you focus on letting go of all barriers.

- As you get excited you will notice that the end of your vagina will squeeze the tip of his penis and form a tight suction around it. He will feel it too. You both will enjoy this sensation.

- The satisfaction from this type of orgasm is very high. You feel a sense of everything that an orgasm is meant to be. Not only do you get a release, but you are fully penetrated by your partner. Ultimately this is part of what you want; to connect at the deepest level. With this type of intercourse, you automatically feel more connected with your lover. Perhaps it was designed that way.

Sexercise: Write about your experience here. How can you improve this technique for next time?

Your Secret Chamber

What was the best way for you to get highly aroused?

What are other ways you want to become aroused?

Positions you tried. What worked best?

Orgasm results

How did the pleasure feel? What did you notice?

What will you try next time?

Now that you have mastered several types of orgasms, practice often. Making love is the highest way that you can connect with your partner.

Intimacy will also open you up to your feminine essence, which is creative energy, nurturing, and enlightening the world. Your time spent in the bedroom will make you a better women and the world a better place to be because your radiance will impact many people for the better.

When you are well practiced, then move on to my book called *Deep Connection*. In this book you will learn many advanced orgasms involving deep penetration. This book focuses on how to take your union with your partner to more profound levels. Increased intimacy creates increased bonding. Not only does your pleasure improve, but so does the closeness between you.

You will learn effective communication techniques regarding intimacy and ways to improve the quality of time that you spend together.

Enjoy this beautiful part of your union. Appreciate your lover and all that you gain from being loved, held and touched. Every aspect of your life is improved by healthy intimacy.

Chapter 10
Don't Get Caught

I can't stress enough how important it is to know the sexual health of your partner. Sexually transmitted disease is a serious threat to your health and safety. Herpes is a life sentence. Syphilis and HIV can be a death sentences. After intercourse is not the time to find out your partner's status.

If you are single and dating new people be direct and open about this issue. Be confident as you ask a man. He should have no reservations about discussing his health with you. You can simply say, "Do you know your status in regards to STD's?" or "Do you know your sexual health? When were you last tested?" If a new partner has never been tested then it is crazy for you to assume that he is clear of all STD's. Many diseases do not have any symptoms, leaving you completely vulnerable to catching something that you don't know your partner has. He may not know that he has a disease or he may be willing to lie just to have sex. Getting an STD can change your life forever.

You can catch any STD from vaginal penetration and from giving oral sex. You can become infected with herpes simply from touching an infected area; penetration is not necessary to spread the disease.

Know your own status as well. Your local Central District Health has affordable testing if you can't afford a doctor. Any of the many STD's are miserable, but some can be life threatening. Herpes can prevent you from ever being with a non-herpes partner.

Use every precaution. Educate yourself about the risks and the symptoms. You might believe that you can't catch herpes unless there is a breakout. That is not true! Doctors were wondering why some people contracted herpes when there was not a break out. They found that people with herpes shed herpes virus cells once a year or more, exposing their partner.

HIV is difficult to transmit. Doctors believe that the virus must be exposed to blood. You can have vaginal bleeding during intercourse, which make you more vulnerable than a man who is much less likely to bleed. There is no need to put yourself at risk. If a man loves you, or cares about you enough to have sex, he should not put you at risk. If he is just a temporary lover who is infected or won't learn his status, find a new partner. Your health is too important. Listen to your intuition!! If something is not adding up, or you see the slightest red flag, don't have sex. Sex should always be a healthy activity. Health and safety first!

Resources

Quick Reference on things to work on:

This page is for a quick reference for you. List here things you want to improve upon which will be ongoing sexercises. You can easily refer back to this page.

1.
2.
3.
4.
5.
6.
7.
8.
9.
10.

Your Secret Chamber

Diana's Seminar:

    Live and e-conference on line. Register at www.yoursecretchamber.com

Diana's websites:

    www.yoursecretchamber.com

    www.dianaanderson.com

Follow her on facebook:

    www.facebook.com/dianaanderson2123

E-mail Diana:

    Diana@dianaanderson.com

Your Secret Chamber

Grab the whole The Venus Method Series:

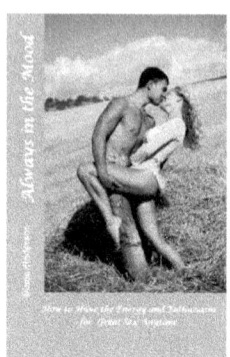

Always in the Mood; A powerful booklet about how to feel ready for your man when he desires you, and enjoy his approach, for great intimacy anytime.

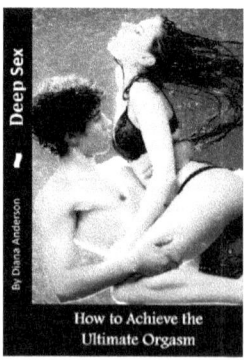

Deep Sex: How to Achieve your Ultimate Orgasm

All orgasms are not created equally. The art of the female climax, long shrouded in mystery and elusive for many women, is made accessible in this down-to-earth, illuminating text. Author and intimacy coach, Diana Anderson presents the essential ingredients and chemistry necessary to achieve advanced orgasmic experience and deep connection with your partner.

http://www.amazon.com/-/e/B00AQ5P61W

Coming soon: *Manifesting with Passion*

Electrify your life goals with the power of Sexual Passion

Your sexual passion is powerful energy which your brain and body respond to. Harness and direct this energy and you have new possibilities at your beckon call. Napoleon Hill said this about sexual passion, "**When driven by this desire, men develop keenness of imagination, courage, will-power, persistence, and creative ability unknown to them at other times.**" (Think and Grow Rich.) Hill failed to tell us how to control this energy. Now the tools to manifest with powers as strong as lust, and climax are

http://www.amazon.com/-/e/B00AQ5P61W

Your Secret Chamber

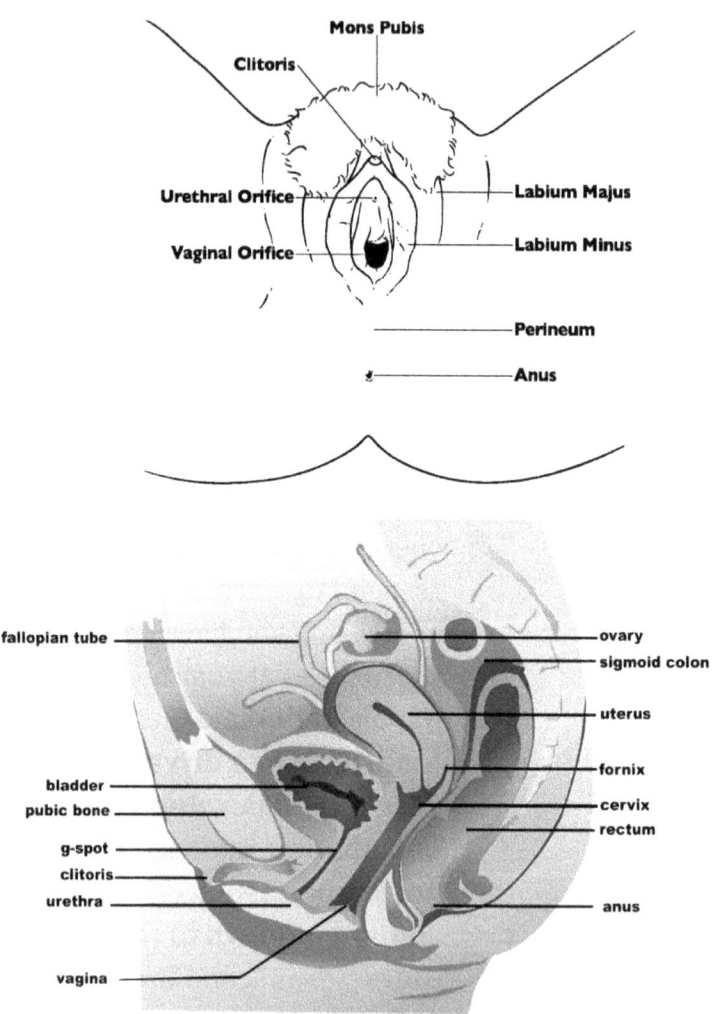

Your Secret Chamber

About the Author:

Diana Anderson writes and coaches women on intimacy and sexuality. *Your Secret Chamber* is a reflection of this work and draws from her own experience building powerful, intimate relationships that improved her as a woman. This book offers a unique, practical approach to opening women, and couples, to their full potential.

Diana's motto is "make every moment count." When she is not writing she is connecting with people through travel and playing outside. A few of her favorite activities include skiing, biking, rafting, golfing and parasailing – having fun and "doing." She has traveled extensively in the US and Europe and escapes to a growing list of tropical islands. Embracing people from all walks of life, Diana channels her experience into expanding the possibilities for everyone.

Her greatest joys are her three daughters and Diana continues to draw inspiration from these three artistic women, her mother and her sister. Born and raised in Idaho, Diana lives in Sun Valley.

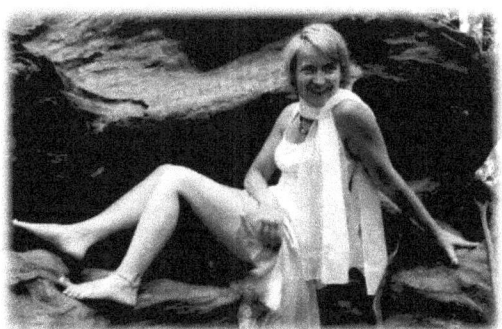

www.ingramcontent.com/pod-product-compliance
Lightning Source LLC
Chambersburg PA
CBHW071502040426
42444CB00008B/1454